SEVENTH EDITION

MOS®

Pharm

Memory

Visual, Mnemonic, &

JoAnn Zerwekh, MSN, EdD, RN
President/CEO
Nursing Education Consultants, Inc.
Chandler, Arizona

Ashley Garneau, PhD, RN
Nursing Faculty
GateWay Community College
Phoenix, Arizona

CJ Miller, BSN, RN
Illustrator
Cedar Rapids, Iowa

REVIEWED BY

Pamela Harvey, MSN, BSN, ASN, RN, BLS
Instructor, Medical Assistant Program
Bradford Union Career Technical Center
Starke, Florida

Robin Ye, RPh, PharmD, BCPS, BLS
Clinical Pharmacist, NorthShore University HealthSystem, Glenbrook Hospital
Glenview, Illinois

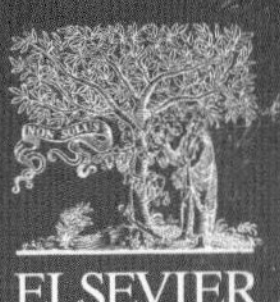

ELSEVIER

Elsevier
3251 Riverport Lane
St. Louis, Missouri 63043

MOSBY'S PHARMACOLOGY MEMORY NOTECARDS,
SEVENTH EDITION ISBN: 978-0-443-11098-6

Notice

Practitioners and researchers must always rely on their own experience and knowledge in evaluating and using any information, methods, compounds or experiments described herein. Because of rapid advances in the medical sciences, in particular, independent verification of diagnoses and drug dosages should be made. To the fullest extent of the law, no responsibility is assumed by Elsevier, authors, editors or contributors for any injury and/or damage to persons or property as a matter of products liability, negligence or otherwise, or from any use or operation of any methods, products, instructions, or ideas contained in the material herein.

Previous editions copyrighted 2022, 2019, 2017, 2015, 2012, and 2008

Senior Content Strategist: Yvonne Alexopoulos
Senior Preceding Content Development Specialist: Rebecca Leenhouts
Publishing Services Manager: Deepthi Unni
Senior Project Manager: Kamatchi Madhavan
Design Direction: Brian Salisbury

Printed in India

Last digit is the print number: 9 8 7 6 5 4 3 2 1

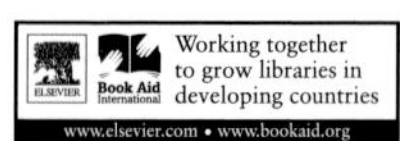

Contents

ADMINISTRATION, 1

ANALGESICS AND NSAIDs, 17

ANTIBIOTICS / ANTIVIRALS / ANTIFUNGALS, 35

CENTRAL NERVOUS SYSTEM, 111

CORTICOSTEROIDS, 123

DIURETICS, 127

ENDOCRINE, 135

EYE AND EAR, 145

REPRODUCTIVE / OBSTETRICS, 199

VITAMINS AND MINERALS, 213

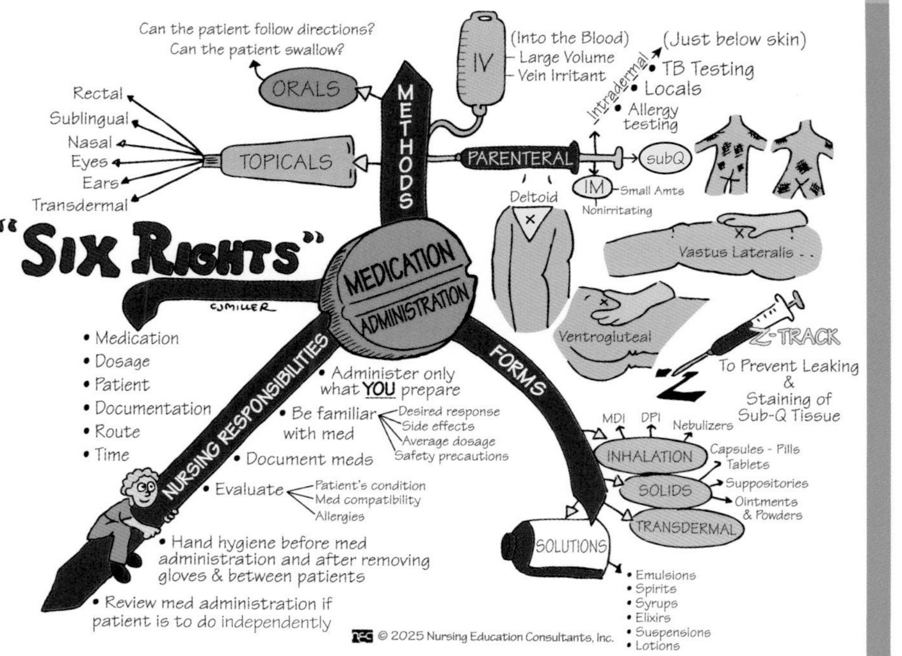
"SIX RIGHTS"
• Medication
• Dosage
• Patient
• Documentation
• Route
• Time
CJMILLER
MEDICATION
ADMINISTRATION
METHODS
ORALS
Can the patient follow directions?
Can the patient swallow?
TOPICALS
Rectal
Sublingual
Nasal
Eyes
Ears
Transdermal
PARENTERAL
IV
(Into the Blood)
Large Volume
Vein Irritant
Intradermal
(Just below skin)
• TB Testing
• Locals
• Allergy testing
subQ
IM
Small Amts
Nonirritating
Deltoid
Ventrogluteal
Vastus Lateralis
Z-TRACK
To Prevent Leaking & Staining of Sub-Q Tissue
FORMS
INHALATION
MDI
DPI
Nebulizers
SOLIDS
Capsules - Pills
Tablets
Suppositories
TRANSDERMAL
Ointments & Powders
SOLUTIONS
• Emulsions
• Spirits
• Syrups
• Elixirs
• Suspensions
• Lotions
NURSING RESPONSIBILITIES
• Administer only what YOU prepare
• Be familiar with med
Desired response
Side effects
Average dosage
Safety precautions
• Document meds
• Evaluate
Patient's condition
Med compatibility
Allergies
• Hand hygiene before med administration and after removing gloves & between patients
• Review med administration if patient is to do independently
© 2025 Nursing Education Consultants, Inc.

What You Need to Know

Medication Administration

SIX RIGHTS OF MEDICATION ADMINISTRATION

- Medication
- Patient
- Route
- Dosage
- Time
- Documentation

ROUTES OF ADMINISTRATION

- Enteral or oral (most common)—ingested into gastrointestinal (GI) tract
- Parenteral—injected into blood or body tissues (intravenous [IV], intramuscular [IM], subcutaneous [subQ])
- Topical (transdermal)—absorbed across skin or mucous membrane
- Inhalation—inhaled directly into lung to elicit local effects
- Rectal and vaginal suppository—inserted for local effects

NURSING IMPLICATIONS

1. Only administer medications you have prepared.
2. Do not document administration of medications until after administration, or after witnessing administration of medications if serving as a second nurse verifier.
3. Read medication label carefully; not all formulations of parenteral medications are appropriate for IV administration (e.g., insulin for IV use).
4. Know your medications.
   - Why is this patient receiving this medication?
   - What nursing observations will tell you the desired medication action is occurring?
   - What are the nursing implications specific to this medication?
5. Do not leave medications at the bedside.
6. Check medication compatibility if administering IV.
7. Medications prepared for one route may differ in concentration for another different route (e.g., subQ epinephrine preparation is concentrated, whereas IV preparation is dilute).
   - Administering a subQ epinephrine preparation IV could be fatal because of an overstimulation of the cardiac system.
8. Use at least two identifiers to determine the correct patient before administering any type of medication (e.g., armband with barcode and date of birth).
9. Have another nurse check medication calculations.
10. IM injections:
    - Do not inject more than 3 mL at one time.
    - Use the smallest gauge needle necessary to administer medication correctly.

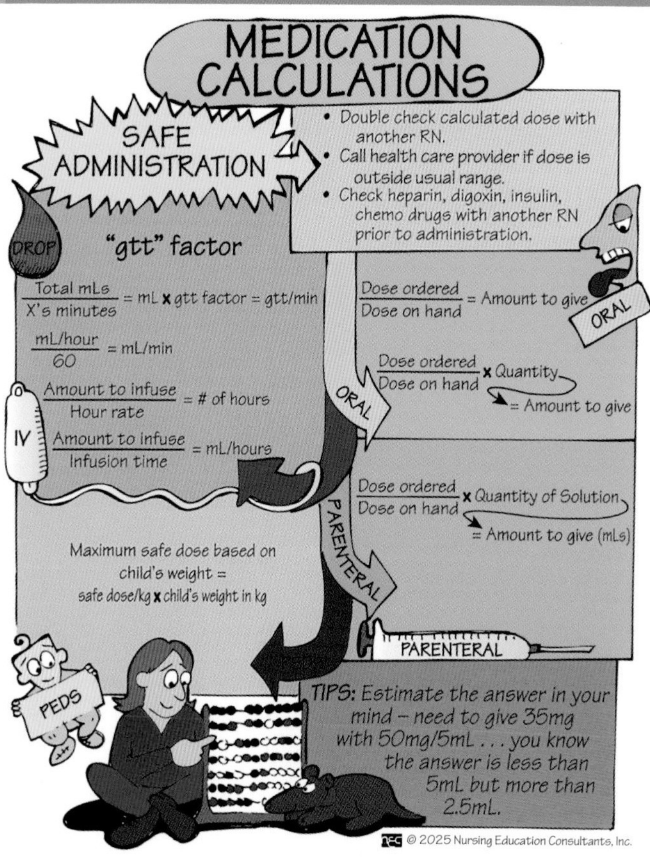
MEDICATION CALCULATIONS
SAFE ADMINISTRATION
• Double check calculated dose with another RN.
• Call health care provider if dose is outside usual range.
• Check heparin, digoxin, insulin, chemo drugs with another RN prior to administration.
DROP
"gtt" factor
Total mLs / X's minutes = mL x gtt factor = gtt/min
mL/hour / 60 = mL/min
Amount to infuse / Hour rate = # of hours
Amount to infuse / Infusion time = mL/hours
IV
Dose ordered / Dose on hand = Amount to give
ORAL
Dose ordered / Dose on hand x Quantity = Amount to give
ORAL
Dose ordered / Dose on hand x Quantity of Solution = Amount to give (mLs)
PARENTERAL
Maximum safe dose based on child's weight = safe dose/kg x child's weight in kg
PARENTERAL
PEDS
TIPS: Estimate the answer in your mind – need to give 35mg with 50mg/5mL . . . you know the answer is less than 5mL but more than 2.5mL.
© 2025 Nursing Education Consultants, Inc.

What You Need to Know

Medication Calculation

METHODS OF CALCULATION

- Drugs requiring individualized dosing can be calculated by body weight (BW) or body surface area (BSA).
- BW and BSA methods are useful when calculating pediatric medications and antineoplastic medications, as well as for patients with low BW, who are obese, or who are older adults.
- Before calculating a dose, all units of measurement should be converted to a single system, preferably what is on the drug label. *For example*: If the medication is supplied in milligrams (mg) and the drug is ordered in grams (g), then convert the g to milligrams (mg).

NURSING IMPLICATIONS

1. Always have another registered nurse (RN) double-check medications when you have to calculate the dosage.
2. Consult the health care provider (HCP) if the dosage is outside the recommended range.
3. Do not administer medications if someone else has calculated the dose for you; administer only those medications that you have calculated and prepared.
4. Be very cautious about calculating drug dosages for pediatric patients.
5. Even when an IV pump for the patient is in place, you still need to know how many milliliters per hour the IV should be infusing. This infusion rate is important to know to set the pump and to check the accuracy of delivery.
6. The West Nomogram uses a child's height and weight to determine the body surface area (BSA). The BSA formula is used to determine the medication dosage for a specific pediatric patient.

Important nursing implications	Serious/life-threatening implications
Most frequent side effects	Patient teaching

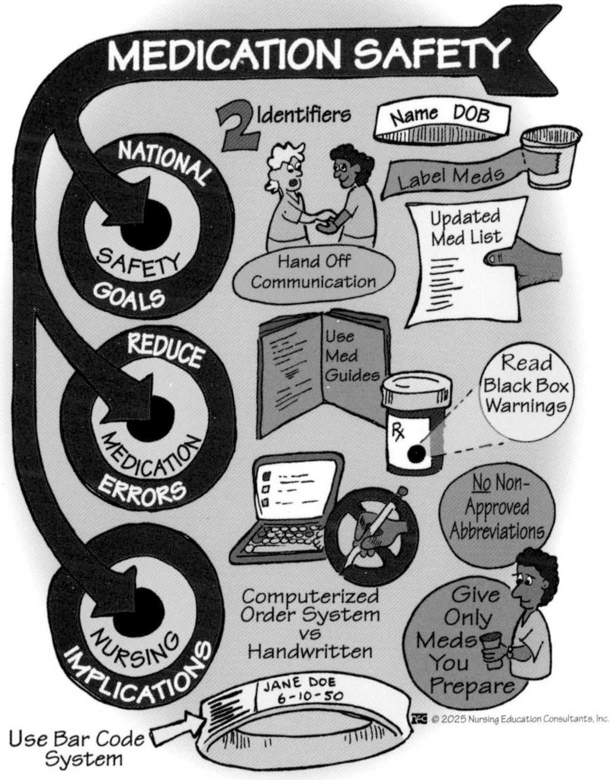
MEDICATION SAFETY
2 Identifiers
Name DOB
Label Meds
Updated Med List
Hand Off Communication
NATIONAL SAFETY GOALS
REDUCE MEDICATION ERRORS
NURSING IMPLICATIONS
Use Med Guides
Read Black Box Warnings
No Non-Approved Abbreviations
Computerized Order System vs Handwritten
Give Only Meds You Prepare
JANE DOE 6-10-50
Use Bar Code System
© 2025 Nursing Education Consultants, Inc.

What You Need to Know

Medication Safety

NATIONAL PATIENT SAFETY GOALS*

- Identify patients correctly using at least two identifiers, such as the patient's name, date of birth, or medical record number.
- Use medications safely, label medications that are not labeled (e.g., medication in syringes), and do this in the area where the medication is prepared.
- Take extra care with patients who take anticoagulant medicines.
- Record and pass along correct information about a patient's medicine. Find out what medicines the patient is taking. Compare those medicines with new medicines given to the patient.
- Give the patient written information about the medicines they need to take.
- Tell the patient it is important to bring an up-to-date list of medicines every time they visit a HCP or health care facility.

REDUCE MEDICATION ERRORS

- Use Medication Guides (MedGuides), which are created to educate patients about how to minimize harm from potentially dangerous drugs.
- Review all *black box warnings* before administering medication.
- The Institute of Medicine identifies three categories of fatal medication errors: human factors (e.g., administering a drug IV instead of IM), communication mistakes (e.g., illegible handwriting of an order), and name confusion (e.g., medications that sound like or look like another medication).

NURSING IMPLICATIONS

1. All high-alert medications should have a safety checklist.
2. Replace handwritten medication orders with a computerized order entry system.
3. Avoid using error-prone abbreviations; see "Do Not Use List" from the Joint Commission.
4. Conduct a medication reconciliation by comparing what medications the patient is currently taking with a list of new medications being prescribed.
5. Use a computerized barcode system that matches the patient's armband barcode to a drug barcode.
6. Administer only medications that you prepare.
7. Have two nurses verify and sign off on high-alert medications (e.g., epinephrine, insulin, chemotherapy).

* National Patient Safety Goals related specifically to medications.

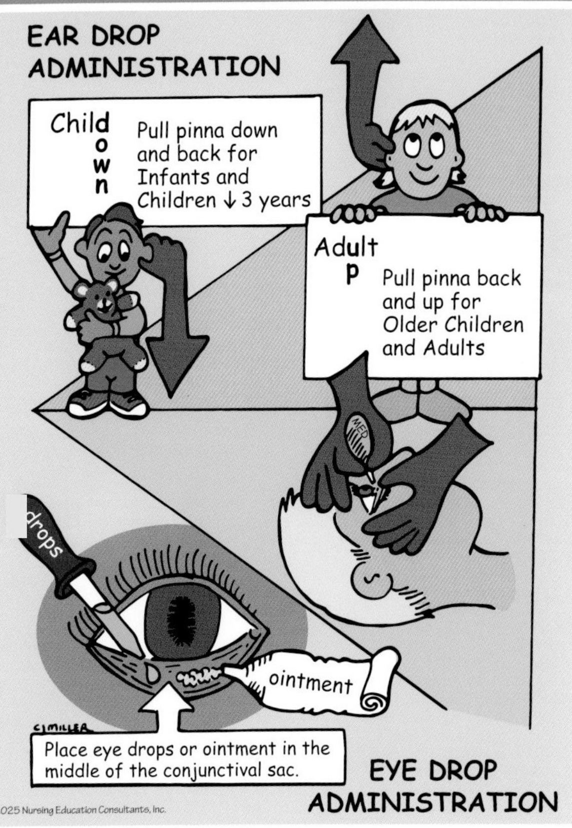
EAR DROP ADMINISTRATION
Child down
Pull pinna down and back for Infants and Children ↓ 3 years
Adult up
Pull pinna back and up for Older Children and Adults
MED
drops
ointment
CJMILLER
Place eye drops or ointment in the middle of the conjunctival sac.
EYE DROP ADMINISTRATION
© 2025 Nursing Education Consultants, Inc.

What You Need to Know

Ear and Eye Drop Administration

EAR DROP PROCEDURE

- Perform hand hygiene and wear gloves.
- Position patient supine on their side with affected ear up.
- Medication should be at least room temperature, not cold.
- Open ear canal of an adult by drawing back on the pinna and slightly upward.
- Open ear canal of a child less than 3 years of age by drawing back on the pinna and slightly downward.
- Allow the prescribed number of drops to fall along the inside of the ear and flow into the ear by gravity. Do not attempt to put the drops directly on the eardrum.
- Have the patient remain supine for 5 minutes to keep the medication from leaking out.

EYE DROP PROCEDURE

- Perform hand hygiene and wear gloves.
- Medication should be at least room temperature, not cold.
- Hold clean cotton ball or tissue in nondominant hand on patient's cheekbone just below lower eyelid.
- Ask patient to look at ceiling and instill eye drop in conjunctival sac.

USES

- Treat ear and eye infections
- Dissolve earwax (cerumen)
- Decrease pain

NURSING IMPLICATIONS

Ear

1. If medication is not instilled at room temperature, the patient may experience vertigo, dizziness, pain, and nausea.
2. If ear drainage is observed, assess patient and determine whether the eardrum is ruptured. If ruptured, do not administer medication until HCP is consulted.
3. Do not occlude ear canal with dropper or syringe.
4. Never force medication into an occluded ear canal; doing so creates pressure, which could damage or rupture the eardrum.

Eye

1. Never press directly against patient's eyeball.
2. When administering drops that have systemic effects, apply gentle pressure to patient's nasolacrimal duct with a clean tissue for 30 to 60 seconds over each eye, one at a time.
3. Avoid touching the eyelids or other eye structures with eyedroppers or ointment tubes to reduce transmitting infection from one eye to the other.
4. Use eye medication only for the patient's affected eye.

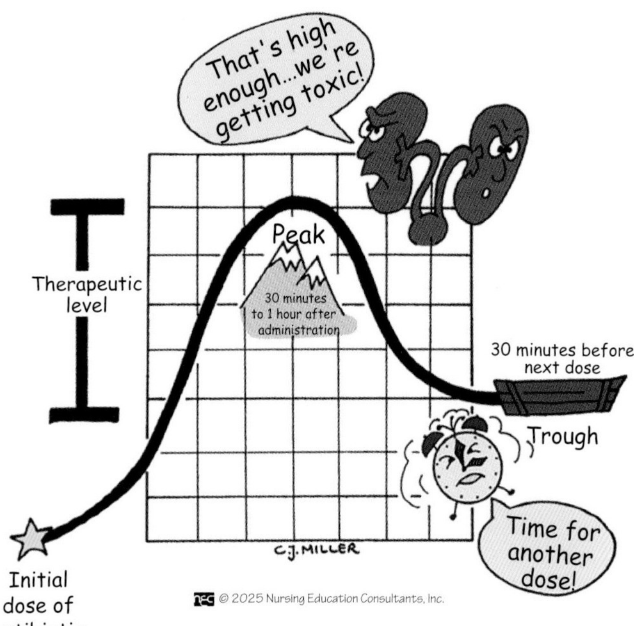
PEAK AND TROUGH
That's high enough...we're getting toxic!
Peak
30 minutes to 1 hour after administration
Therapeutic level
30 minutes before next dose
Trough
Time for another dose!
Initial dose of antibiotic
C.J. MILLER
© 2025 Nursing Education Consultants, Inc.

What You Need to Know

Peak and Trough

USES

- It is primarily used to monitor levels of the aminoglycoside family of antibiotics. Monitoring serum drug levels enables the HCP to individualize dosage levels to maximal effectiveness, which allows drug levels to be at an effective but not toxic level.
- If the patient is on a once-daily dose, the HCP will often focus on the *trough* level instead of the *peak* level. The serum level of the medication must drop down to a designated level. One daily dose means that the highest peak level is guaranteed when the daily dose is given.
- When multiple daily doses are given, both peak and trough levels must be measured. The timing of the levels drawn is important for accuracy.
- The peak level (highest blood level of drug) is usually 1 to 3 hours after oral administration. Levels are usually drawn 30 minutes to 1 hour after an IM injection, 30 minutes after completion of an IV infusion, or at the drug's proposed peak time.
- If the patient is taking multiple doses, the trough sample (lowest blood level of drug) should be taken just before the next dose.

NURSING IMPLICATIONS

1. If the trough level is too high, toxicity can occur. Nephrotoxicity and ototoxicity are the primary problems of aminoglycosides.
2. If the peak is too low, no or minimal therapeutic effect is achieved.
3. Check laboratory values for peak and trough levels.
4. Report serum levels that are not within established ranges of peak and trough levels.
5. Explain to the patient the purpose for measurement of peak and trough levels.
6. Maintain accuracy of values; ensure that serum laboratory values are drawn at scheduled times.
7. Risk of toxicity is increased in patients with decreased kidney function.

Important nursing implications	Serious/life-threatening implications
Most frequent side effects	Patient teaching

GUIDE TO DRUG OVERDOSE

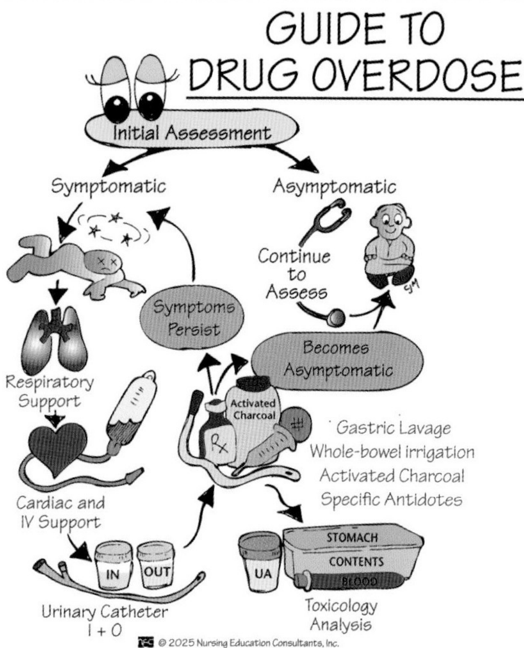

What You Need to Know

Guide to Drug Overdose

NURSING MANAGEMENT

1. Make an initial assessment, including vital signs and level of consciousness.
2. The specific drug taken in the overdose will dictate the treatment.
   - Obtain information about the amount of drug, time, and underlying medical problems.
   - Direct family member or other individual to bring drug and/or container to the emergency department.
   - If depressant drug effects are present, naloxone and flumazenil may be administered, because naloxone counteracts the opiate effects and flumazenil reverses the effects of benzodiazepine overdose.
3. Perform gastric lavage to remove unabsorbed drugs mechanically from the stomach.
4. Activated charcoal may be given to help bind drugs taken orally while still in the GI tract.
   - Activated charcoal reduces the amount of drug absorbed into the blood.
   - The drug, bound to the charcoal, is then expelled in the stool.
5. Whole-bowel irrigation with polyethylene glycol (GoLYTELY) administered over a 5-hour period is used for ingestion of iron, lithium, and lead along with sustained-release medications.
6. Respiratory and cardiac support may be required for symptomatic cases.
7. IV lines, laboratory tests for toxicologic analysis, and a urinary catheter may also be ordered.

Helpful mnemonic for opiate overdose:
Cool to the touch and unresponsive to pain.
Hunger diminished and scars over vein.
Pupils pinpointed and blood pressure low.
Urine diminished and breathing slow.

Another mnemonic to help you remember the most rapid (speedy) way toxins or medications enter the body:
4 **S**'s—Stick it, **S**niff it, **S**uck it, **S**oak it
Stick: injection; **S**niff: inhalation; **S**uck: ingestion; **S**oak: absorption

Important nursing implications	Serious/life-threatening implications
Most frequent side effects	Patient teaching

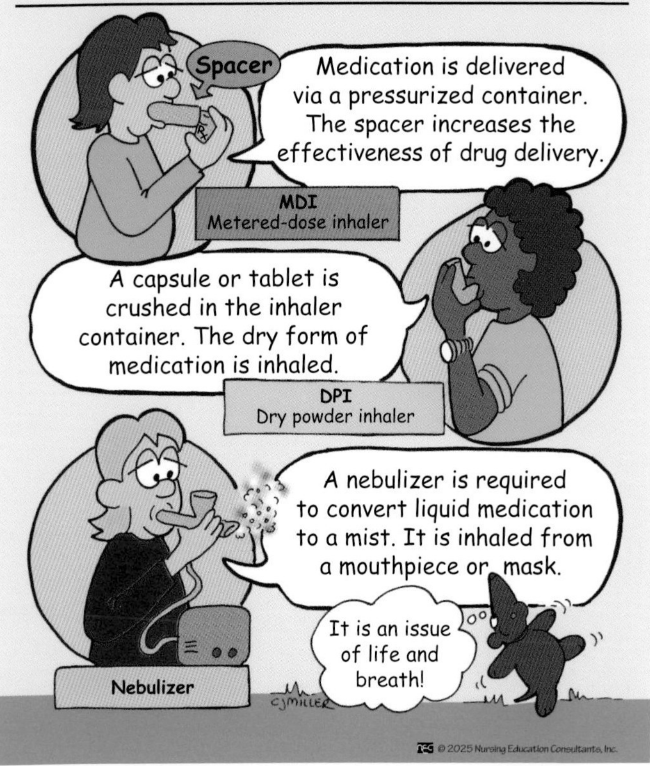
ADMINISTRATION OF MEDICATIONS BY INHALATION
Spacer
Medication is delivered via a pressurized container. The spacer increases the effectiveness of drug delivery.
MDI
Metered-dose inhaler
A capsule or tablet is crushed in the inhaler container. The dry form of medication is inhaled.
DPI
Dry powder inhaler
A nebulizer is required to convert liquid medication to a mist. It is inhaled from a mouthpiece or mask.
It is an issue of life and breath!
Nebulizer
CJMILLER
© 2025 Nursing Education Consultants, Inc.

What You Need to Know

Administration of Medications by Inhalation

METERED-DOSE INHALER

- Hand-held pressurized containers deliver a measured dose of medication with each "puff."
- Dosing may require two "puffs"—patient should wait 1 minute between "puffs."
- A spacer device may be used to increase the delivery of medication and to decrease medication deposited in the mouth and throat. Pediatric patients often require a spacer.
- Requires "hand-lung coordination"—patient should exhale and, on beginning of inhalation, activate the metered-dose inhaler (MDI).
- Patient should hold their breath for approximately 10 seconds after inhalation.

DRY POWDER INHALER

- Each medication comes with a delivery system. Medication should be administered only with the delivery system provided. No aerosol propellant is used.
- Capsules and tablets are to be administered by inhalation only; medications *are not to be taken by mouth*.
- Delivery system crushes the medication to a fine powder to be inhaled.
- After the system is loaded, teach patient to cover mouthpiece and inhale deeply.
- Compared with MDIs, medication delivery is significantly more efficient.

SMALL-VOLUME NEBULIZER

- A small machine converts a medication solution to a nebulized or mist form.
- The prescribed amount of medication is added to a nebulizer cup or container and attached to the machine.
- Determining whether a diluent needs to be added to the medication to facilitate the delivery is important.
- The most effective method of delivery is via mouthpiece; however, medication may also be delivered via face mask.
- When the mist begins to form at the end of the mouthpiece, ask patient to seal their mouth over the mouthpiece and start a slow, deep breath; patient should hold their breath for a short time and then exhale slowly.
- The mouth should be rinsed after treatment, and equipment should be rinsed and allowed to dry. Do not store wet equipment.
- With inhaled steroid medications, the mouth should be rinsed to prevent infections.

TRANSDERMAL MEDICATION ADMINISTRATION

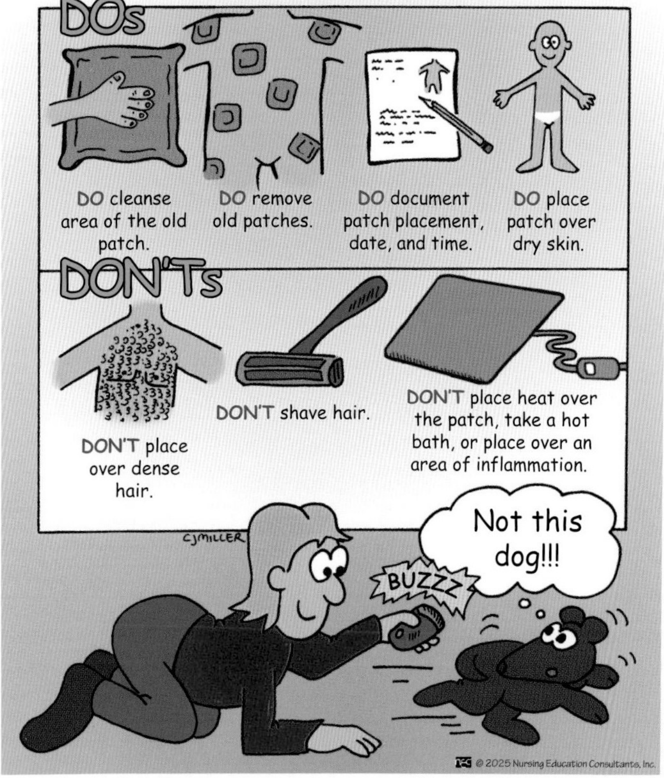

DOs

DO cleanse area of the old patch.

DO remove old patches.

DO document patch placement, date, and time.

DO place patch over dry skin.

DON'Ts

DON'T place over dense hair.

DON'T shave hair.

DON'T place heat over the patch, take a hot bath, or place over an area of inflammation.

CJMILLER

BUZZZ

Not this dog!!!

What You Need to Know

Transdermal Medication Administration

GENERAL

- Transdermal medications are administered topically and absorbed through the skin into the blood; they can exert a systemic effect.
- Avoids first-pass metabolism and decreases bioavailability of medication.
- Provides a controlled, constant release of medication.
- Patients who are obese or diaphoretic may have difficulty absorbing the medication.
- If a patient is going to have a magnetic resonance imaging (MRI) procedure, make sure the patch of transdermal medication does not contain a metallic component. The US Food and Drug Administration recommends that health care professionals note the presence of a patch when they refer patients for an MRI. The patch may be removed before the MRI and replaced after the exam is completed.
- Heat increases the absorption of transdermal medications. Check with the HCP before administering a medication patch to a patient who has a temperature higher than 102°F (38.9°C).
- Do not apply any heat over patch; doing so will increase absorption of medication.
- Do not allow medication to come in direct contact with fingers.

ADMINISTRATION GUIDELINES

1. Follow principles of safe medication administration.
2. Apply patch to dry, hairless area of skin—preferably the chest, abdomen, or upper back.
3. Remove the old patch and cleanse the area; apply a new patch in a different area.
4. Do not apply a patch over an area of emaciated skin or on an area with irritated or broken skin.
5. Do not apply an adhesive dressing over the patch.
6. Dispose of old patches according to facility guidelines. Of specific concern is proper disposal of fentanyl patches.

Important nursing implications

Serious/life-threatening implications

Most frequent side effects

Patient teaching

MORPHINE SULFATE

The opium poppy is one of nature's ways of controlling pain.

Opium Poppy

Morphine Sulfate

C J MILLER

Most common drug for PCA—maintains even pain control.

I didn't know that, but I do know the route can be PO (TAB-LIQ), IV, IM, subQ, rectal, epidural, or intrathecal.

Side effects:

- Decreased blood pressure
- Respiratory depression
- Urinary retention
- Constipation

What You Need to Know

Morphine Sulfate

CLASSIFICATION

Analgesic, opioid agonist ■ Black Box Warning ▲ High Alert

ACTIONS

Interacts at a specific receptor-binding site. Agonist activity at the receptor site can result in analgesia, euphoria, depression, hallucinations, miosis, and sedation. Alters pain at the spinal cord and higher levels in the central nervous system (CNS) (Schedule II on Controlled Substances Act). With prolonged use, the drug produces tolerance and physical dependence.

USES

- Relieves moderate-to-severe pain
- Decreases anxiety and therefore decreases myocardial oxygen demands with pain from a myocardial infarction (MI)

CONTRAINDICATIONS

- Hypersensitivity

PRECAUTIONS

- Severe respiratory depression, seizures, asthma
- Intracranial pressure and suspected head injuries; may mask the development of increased intracranial pressure (IICP)
- Hepatic and kidney dysfunction; biliary tract surgery
- Labor and delivery; may suppress uterine contractions and cause respiratory depression in neonates

SIDE EFFECTS

- Respiratory depression, cough suppression, orthostatic hypotension
- Urinary retention, confusion, constipation, nausea, vomiting
- Tolerance and physical dependency with long-term use
- Toxicity: coma, respiratory depression, pinpoint pupils

NURSING IMPLICATIONS

1. Perform strict documentation and inventory assessment of opioids.
2. Assess pain and vital signs (especially respirations) before and after the dose; do not administer if respirations are less than 12 breaths per minute.
3. Infants and older adults are very sensitive to respiratory depression.
4. Naloxone reverses the effect of morphine.
5. Medication of choice for patient-controlled analgesia.
6. Patients with cancer should receive opioids on a fixed schedule; tolerance may occur, requiring dosage escalation.

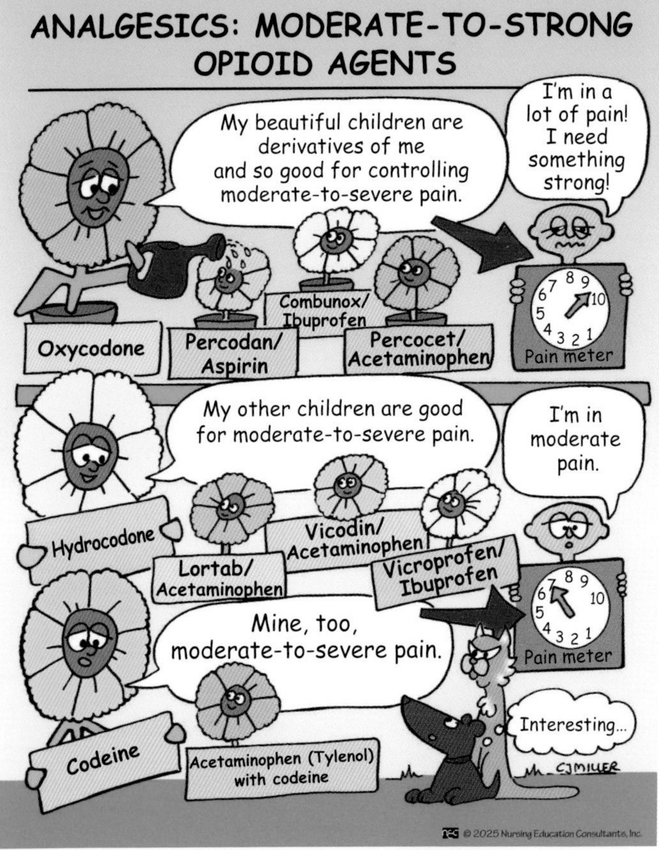
ANALGESICS: MODERATE-TO-STRONG OPIOID AGENTS
My beautiful children are derivatives of me and so good for controlling moderate-to-severe pain.
I'm in a lot of pain! I need something strong!
Oxycodone
Percodan/ Aspirin
Combunox/ Ibuprofen
Percocet/ Acetaminophen
Pain meter
My other children are good for moderate-to-severe pain.
I'm in moderate pain.
Hydrocodone
Lortab/ Acetaminophen
Vicodin/ Acetaminophen
Vicroprofen/ Ibuprofen
Pain meter
Mine, too, moderate-to-severe pain.
Codeine
Acetaminophen (Tylenol) with codeine
Interesting...
CJMILLER
© 2025 Nursing Education Consultants, Inc.

What You Need to Know

Analgesics: Moderate-to-Strong Opioid Agents

ACTIONS ■ Black Box Warning

Bind with receptors in the brain and spinal cord that are associated with pain. Moderate-to-strong opioid analgesics are similar to morphine; however, pain control is less effective and the potential for respiratory depression is less.

OPIOID ANALGESICS

Oxycodone—PO, Schedule II

- **Percodan**—combined with aspirin
- **Percocet, Roxicet, Tylox**—combined with acetaminophen
- **Combunox**—combined with ibuprofen
- **OxyContin**—controlled release, dosing is usually every 12 hours with another analgesic for breakthrough pain

Hydrocodone—PO, Schedule II

- **Lortab**—combined with acetaminophen
- **Vicodin**—combined with acetaminophen
- **Vicoprofen**—combined with ibuprofen
- May also be combined with antihistamines and nasal decongestants for cough suppression

Codeine—PO, Schedule II

- Acetaminophen with codeine (PO)
- Frequently combined with various agents for suppression of cough

NURSING IMPLICATIONS

1. Assessment is critical to effective pain control. Carefully assess patient's level of pain and administer analgesic as ordered.
2. Follow institution procedure for administering an opioid (Controlled Substance Act).
3. Reassess the patient 1 hour after administering medication.
4. Administer medication before pain returns; fixed schedule of dosing may be more efficient than "as needed" dosing for the first 24 hours postoperatively.
5. Developing physical dependence is rare for hospitalized patients who receive short-term therapy for pain. Even when physical dependence does occur, patients rarely develop addictive behavior; the majority go through a gradual withdrawal and never take opioids again.

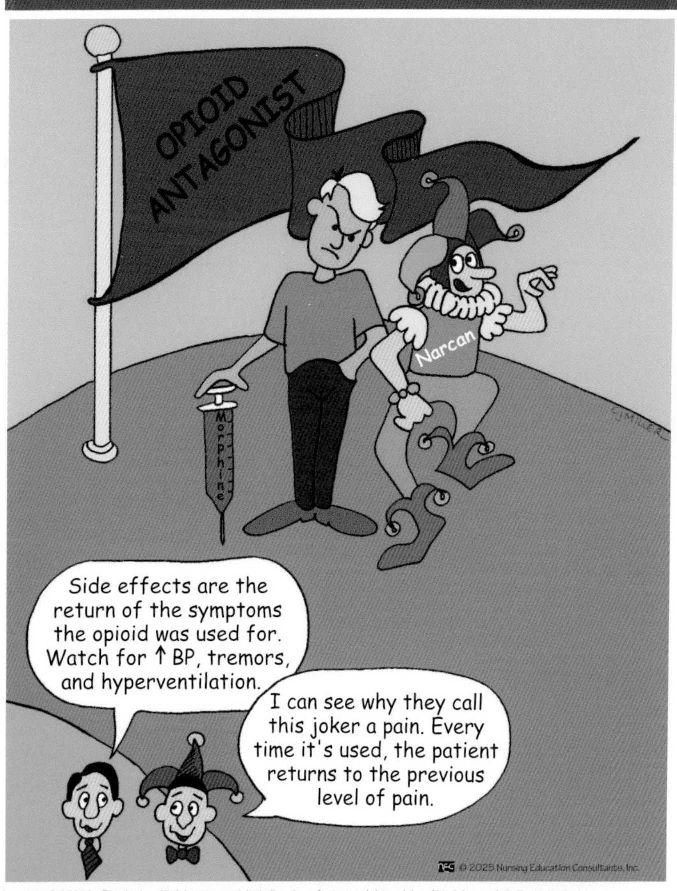
OPIOID ANTAGONIST
Narcan
Morphine
Side effects are the return of the symptoms the opioid was used for. Watch for ↑ BP, tremors, and hyperventilation.
I can see why they call this joker a pain. Every time it's used, the patient returns to the previous level of pain.
© 2025 Nursing Education Consultants, Inc.

What You Need to Know

Opioid Antagonists: Naloxone (Narcan)

ACTIONS

Opioid antagonists block (or antagonize) opiate receptor sites. Its principal use is the treatment of opioid overdose.

USES

- Reverse the opiate effects of narcotic overdose and respiratory depression

CONTRAINDICATIONS AND PRECAUTIONS

- Patients who are using nonopioid drugs
- Neonates and children
- Patients with a history of dependency; may precipitate acute withdrawal

SIDE EFFECTS

- Too rapid reversal of opioid overdose—nausea, vomiting, tremors, hypertension
- Minimal pharmacologic effects in the absence of narcotics
- Reversal of analgesia

NURSING IMPLICATIONS

1. The preferred route of administration is intravenous (IV); response is within 1 to 2 minutes, and peak action is within 20 to 60 minutes.
2. Patient should be frequently assessed; if the opioid analgesic lasts longer in the system than the action of the naloxone, then respiratory depression may recur.
3. If a patient has a history of opioid dependency, administration of naloxone may produce symptoms of acute withdrawal.
4. If accidental poisoning or possible opioid overdose is a concern, naloxone is usually administered.
5. Not effective against barbiturates or other CNS depressants.
6. Assess for increased pain with reversal of opiate in the postoperative patient.

Important nursing implications | Serious/life-threatening implications

Most frequent side effects | Patient teaching

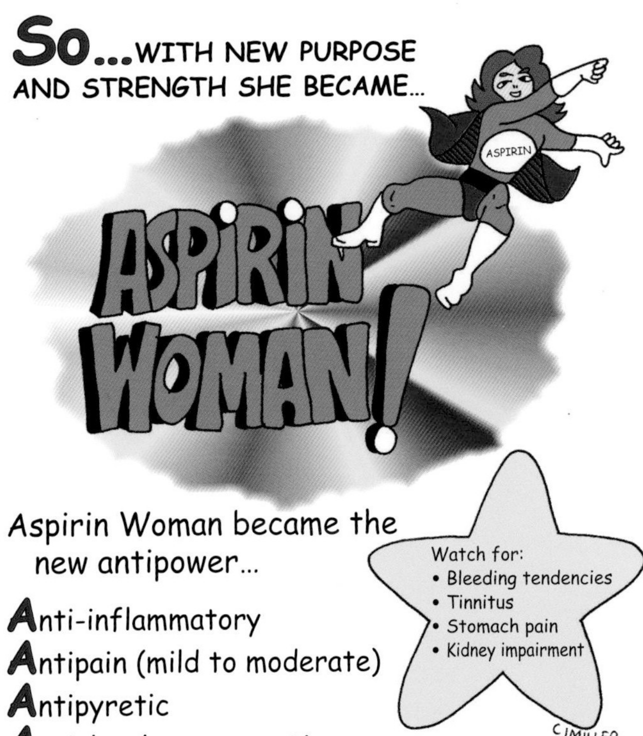
So...WITH NEW PURPOSE
AND STRENGTH SHE BECAME...
ASPIRIN
ASPIRIN WOMAN!
Aspirin Woman became the new antipower...
Anti-inflammatory
Antipain (mild to moderate)
Antipyretic
Antiplatelet aggregation
Watch for:
• Bleeding tendencies
• Tinnitus
• Stomach pain
• Kidney impairment
CJMILLER

What You Need to Know

Acetylsalicylic Acid—Aspirin

CLASSIFICATION

Analgesic, antipyretic, antiplatelet; first-generation nonsteroidal anti-inflammatory drug (NSAID) ▲ **High Alert**

ACTIONS

It is a nonselective cyclooxygenase (COX) inhibitor that decreases the formation of prostaglandins involved in the production of inflammation, pain, and fever. Inhibits platelet aggregation.

USES

- Relieves low-to-moderate pain
- Decreases inflammation in systemic lupus erythematosus, rheumatoid arthritis, osteoarthritis, bursitis, tendonitis
- Is a prophylactic medication to reduce the risk of transient ischemic attack, ischemic stroke, MI

CONTRAINDICATIONS AND PRECAUTIONS

- Hypersensitivity to salicylates
- Do not use during pregnancy
- Do not administer to children younger than 18 years of age; increased risk of Reye syndrome
- History of gastrointestinal (GI) ulceration, peptic ulcer disease, or any bleeding disorders

SIDE EFFECTS

- Decreases platelet aggregation; increases bleeding, potential bruising
- Epigastric distress, heartburn, nausea
- Aspirin overdose or toxicity—respiratory alkalosis that progresses to respiratory depression and acidosis; hyperthermia, sweating, dehydration with electrolyte imbalance; tinnitus; headache

NURSING IMPLICATIONS

1. Teach patient to take with milk or full glass of water to decrease gastric irritation.
2. Teach safety measures to parents regarding medications at home.
3. The potential for toxicity is high in older adults and children.
4. Teach patient to avoid concurrent use of alcohol to decrease GI irritation.
5. Explain that patient should not take aspirin for at least 1 week before surgery.
6. Evaluate patient to determine the purpose of medication—pain, inflammation, or antiplatelet action.
7. Antiplatelet effect persists for about 8 days (life span of a platelet).

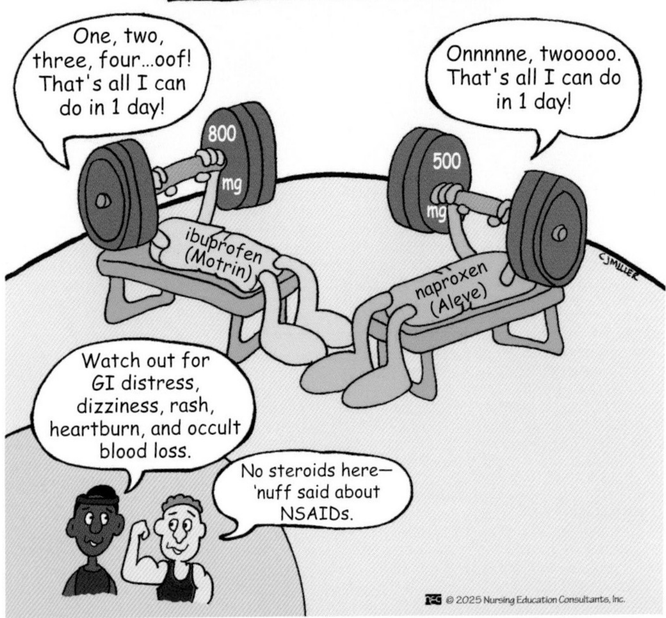
NSAID GYM
NO PAIN, NO FLAME, AND NO HEAT WHEN WE MEET
(ANALGESIC, ANTI-INFLAMMATORY, ANTIPYRETIC)
One, two, three, four...oof! That's all I can do in 1 day!
Onnnnne, twooooo. That's all I can do in 1 day!
800 mg
500 mg
ibuprofen (Motrin)
naproxen (Aleve)
Watch out for GI distress, dizziness, rash, heartburn, and occult blood loss.
No steroids here—'nuff said about NSAIDs.
© 2025 Nursing Education Consultants, Inc.

What You Need to Know

First-Generation NSAIDs—Nonaspirin

ACTIONS

Suppress inflammation by inhibiting both COX-1 and COX-2 enzymes that are responsible for the synthesis of prostaglandins. NSAIDs inhibit the formation and release of prostaglandin. ■ Black Box Warning

EXAMPLES OF FIRST-GENERATION NSAIDs

Ibuprofen (e.g., Motrin, Advil), naproxen (Aleve), indomethacin (Indocin), piroxicam (Feldene), meloxicam (Mobic), and numerous others

USES

- Primary use is for rheumatoid arthritis and osteoarthritis
- Reduce inflammation and pain of dysmenorrhea, bursitis, tendonitis
- Decrease fever

CONTRAINDICATIONS AND PRECAUTIONS

- History of GI inflammation, ulceration, bleeding
- Not recommended for use during pregnancy
- Do not take before or for 14 days after coronary artery bypass graft surgery
- Can cause increased risk of renal insufficiency in older patients with other chronic conditions

SIDE EFFECTS

- Dyspepsia, anorexia, nausea, vomiting, fluid retention
- Rash, dizziness, heartburn, GI bleeding

NURSING IMPLICATIONS

1. Take with food or milk to reduce GI distress.
2. Instruct patient to use correct concentrations for age group (e.g., infants, children).
3. Do not crush or chew enteric-coated tablets.
4. Teach patient to avoid alcohol and aspirin products while taking NSAIDs.
5. Patient should avoid all NSAIDs for at least 1 week before surgery or invasive diagnostics.
6. Nonaspirin NSAIDs do not protect against MI and stroke, like aspirin does; in fact, they increase the risk of thrombotic events, with risk being the highest with indomethacin (Indocin), sulindac (Clinoril), and meloxicam (Mobic).
7. If patient is also taking aspirin, administer NSAIDs 2 hours after aspirin administration.

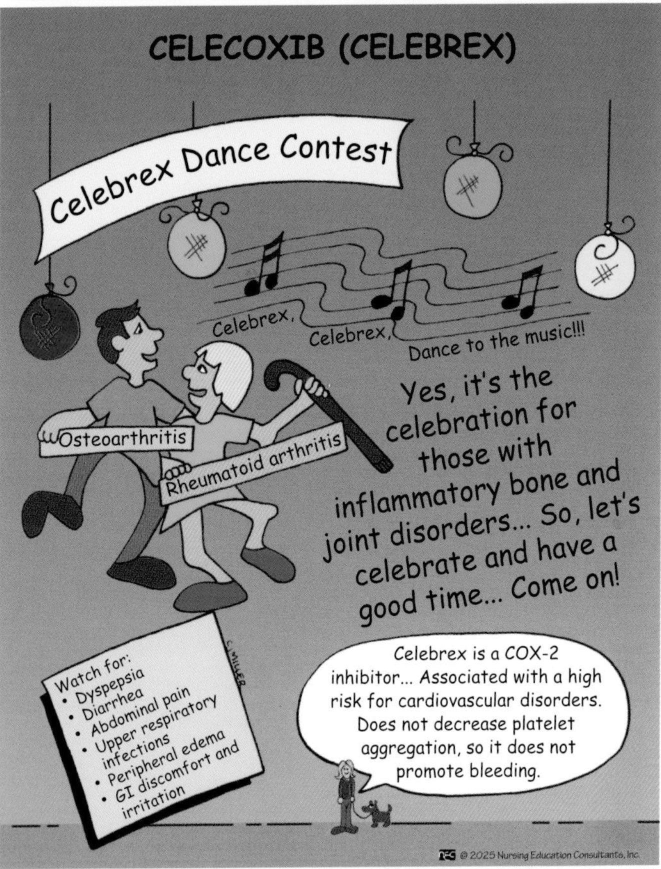
CELECOXIB (CELEBREX)
Celebrex Dance Contest
Celebrex,
Celebrex,
Dance to the music!!!
Yes, it's the celebration for those with inflammatory bone and joint disorders... So, let's celebrate and have a good time... Come on!
Osteoarthritis
Rheumatoid arthritis
Watch for:
• Dyspepsia
• Diarrhea
• Abdominal pain
• Upper respiratory infections
• Peripheral edema
• GI discomfort and irritation
C. MILLER
Celebrex is a COX-2 inhibitor... Associated with a high risk for cardiovascular disorders. Does not decrease platelet aggregation, so it does not promote bleeding.
© 2025 Nursing Education Consultants, Inc.

What You Need to Know

Second-Generation NSAIDs (COX-2 Inhibitor or Coxibs)

CLASSIFICATION

Analgesic, anti-inflammatory; NSAID ■ Black Box Warning

ACTION

Celecoxib (Celebrex) inhibits prostaglandin synthesis by selectively inhibiting COX-2, an enzyme needed for biosynthesis, which suppresses pain and inflammation while posing a lower risk of gastric ulceration.

USES

- Relieves low-to-moderate pain
- Decreases inflammation in systemic lupus erythematosus, rheumatoid arthritis, osteoarthritis

CONTRAINDICATIONS AND PRECAUTIONS

- May increase the risk of MI, stroke, other serious cardiovascular events
- Do not use during pregnancy, especially the third trimester
- Can impair kidney function
- Can precipitate an allergic reaction in patients allergic to sulfonamides
- Do not use in patients with a history of hypertension, edema, heart failure, or kidney disease

SIDE EFFECTS

- Dyspepsia, abdominal pain, fatigue, nervousness, and paresthesia
- Does not decrease platelet aggregation; hence, does not promote bleeding

NURSING IMPLICATIONS

1. Give with milk or a full glass of water to enhance absorption.
2. Do not break, crush, chew, or dissolve caps. Caps can be opened into applesauce or soft food but must be ingested immediately with water.
3. Teach patient to avoid concurrent use of alcohol to decrease GI irritation.
4. Monitor for GI irritation, bleeding episodes, or kidney impairment.
5. Evaluate patient to determine the purpose of medication—reduction in pain and inflammation.
6. Teach patient to avoid the use of NSAIDs to prevent vaccination-associated fever and pain as they may blunt the immune response to the vaccine.

Important nursing implications | Serious/life-threatening implications

Most frequent side effects | Patient teaching

ACETAMINOPHEN

A – Has **analgesic** and **antipyretic** properties.

C – Can blunt the immune response to **childhood** vaccines.

E – Adverse **effects** are rare with a therapeutic dose.

T – **Teach** the patient to avoid ingesting alcohol.

A – **Antidote** is acetylcysteine (Mucomyst).

M – **May** cause hypertension in people who take 500 mg or more per day.

I – **Injury** to the liver may occur with an overdose.

N – Has **no** anti-inflammatory or antirheumatic actions.

O – Maximum **oral** dose for adults is 4000 mg/day.

P – **Precautions** are with pregnancy, breast-feeding, and alcohol use.

H – **Has** the ability to increase the risk of bleeding in those who take warfarin (Coumadin).

E – **Educate** the patient that it can be taken with food or milk.

N – **No** evidence suggests that it causes Reye syndrome.

What You Need to Know

Acetaminophen (Tylenol)

CLASSIFICATION

Analgesic, antipyretic ■ Black Box Warning

ACTIONS

Decreases prostaglandin synthesis in the CNS and has antipyretic and analgesic action. Does not possess anti-inflammatory properties, does not cause gastric ulceration, and does not suppress platelet aggregation or impair kidney blood flow or function.

USES

- Relieves low-to-moderate pain and fever
- Arthralgia, dental pain, dysmenorrhea, headache
- Preferred drug for children having chickenpox or influenza (not associated with Reye syndrome)

CONTRAINDICATIONS AND PRECAUTIONS

- Hypersensitivity
- Precaution during pregnancy and breast-feeding
- Excessive alcohol ingestion
- Liver disease

SIDE EFFECTS

- Adverse effects rare at therapeutic doses
- Overdose or toxicity leads to liver damage

NURSING IMPLICATIONS

1. Give with milk or full glass of water to decrease GI irritation.
2. Teach parents that drug may blunt the immune response to childhood vaccines and should not be given to treat vaccination-associated pain or fever.
3. Teach patient to avoid concurrent use of alcohol to prevent liver damage.
4. Evaluate patient to determine the purpose of medication—pain or fever.
5. Antidote for overdose is acetylcysteine (Mucomyst).
6. If patient is taking warfarin (Coumadin), concurrent use of acetaminophen can increase the risk of bleeding.
7. Monitor medications that may contain acetaminophen so as not to exceed maximum recommended dose.

Important nursing implications	Serious/life-threatening implications
Most frequent side effects	Patient teaching

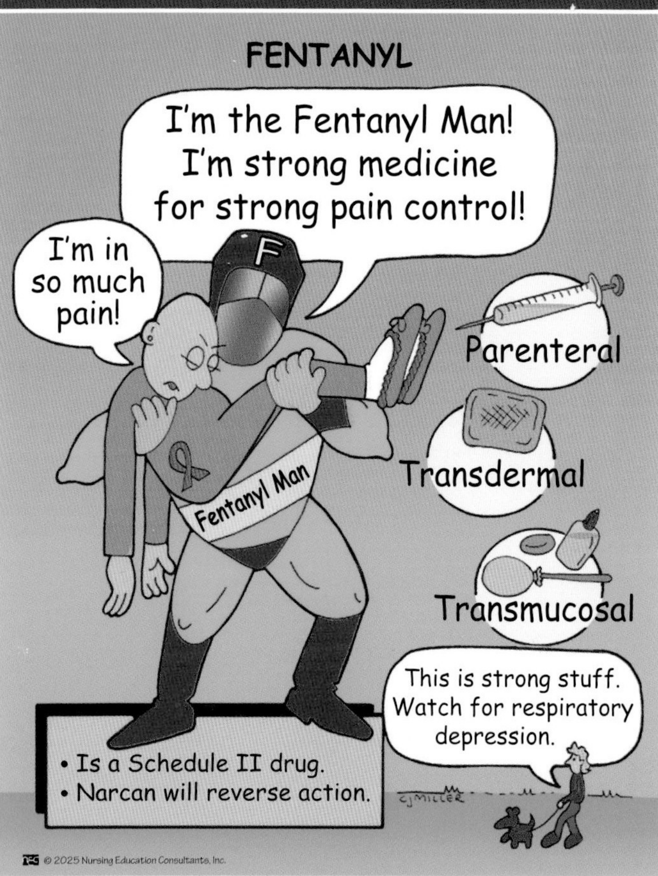
FENTANYL
I'm the Fentanyl Man! I'm strong medicine for strong pain control!
I'm in so much pain!
F
Fentanyl Man
Parenteral
Transdermal
Transmucosal
This is strong stuff. Watch for respiratory depression.
• Is a Schedule II drug.
• Narcan will reverse action.
CJ MILLER
© 2025 Nursing Education Consultants, Inc.

What You Need to Know

Fentanyl

CLASSIFICATION

Strong narcotic analgesic; Schedule II of Controlled Substances Act ■ Black Box Warning ▲ High Alert

USES

- Fentanyl (IM, IV)—facilitates the induction of anesthesia; may be used with droperidol
- Transdermal patches (Duragesic)—relief of persistent pain is reported in patients who are tolerant of opioid agents
- Transdermal iontophoretic system (Ionsys)—a self-contained credit card–sized device that is a needle-free patient-activated system for on-demand delivery
- Transmucosal (lozenge on a stick [Actiq]; buccal tablets [Fentora]; sublingual tablets [Abstral]; sublingual spray [Subsys])
- Intranasal spray (Lazanda)—breakthrough pain in patients with cancer who are opioid tolerant

CONTRAINDICATIONS

- Only indicated for the relief of severe pain
- In patients with suspected head injuries, fentanyl may mask the development of IICP

SIDE EFFECTS

- Respiratory depression
- Sedation, dizziness, euphoria, constipation
- Hypotension, pupillary miosis, urinary retention, nausea
- Tolerance and physical dependency with long-term use

NURSING IMPLICATIONS

1. Perform strict documentation and inventory assessment of opioid.
2. Assess pain and vital signs (especially respirations) before and after the dose; do not administer if respirations are less than 12 breaths per minute.
3. Pay close attention to guidelines for administration.
4. Patch is used for opioid-tolerant patients, not for the control of postoperative pain.
5. Advise patient to store medication(s) out of reach of children.
6. Respiratory depression can be reversed with naloxone (Narcan).
7. Teach patients to avoid exposing the patch to external heat sources (e.g., heating pads, hot baths, electric blankets); doing so can accelerate the release of the medication, as can fever, sunbathing, and strenuous exercise.
8. Teach patient that if intranasal spray has not been used within 5 days, the bottle should be reprimed by spraying once and/or discarded and replaced with a new one.

SALICYLATE (ASPIRIN) POISONING

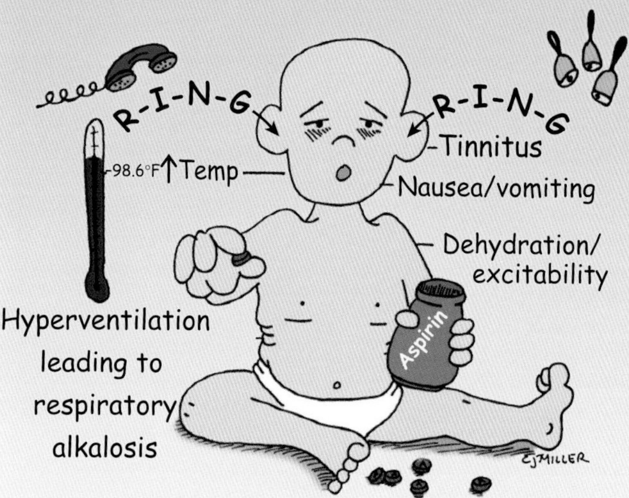

Severe toxicity =

- Metabolic acidosis
- Seizures

Salicylate level greater than 100 mg/dL is severe toxicity.

What You Need to Know

Salicylate (Aspirin) Poisoning

PATHOPHYSIOLOGY ▲ High Alert

Initially, respiratory excitation occurs, producing respiratory alkalosis. As toxicity occurs, respiratory depression occurs, resulting in an increase in carbon dioxide levels, which produces respiratory acidosis. Respiratory acidosis is uncompensated because the bicarbonate stores are depleted during the early stages of poisoning. Metabolic acidosis results from the acidity of aspirin, along with an increased production of lactic and pyruvic acids.

SIGNS AND SYMPTOMS

- Initial symptoms: tinnitus, sweating, headache, and dizziness
- Toxicity: hyperthermia, sweating, and dehydration; respiratory depression, resulting in respiratory acidosis, stupor, and coma
  - Lethal dose for adults is 20 to 25 gm; as little as 4000 mg (4 gm) can be lethal for a child
  - Severe toxicity (salicylate levels >100 mg/dL)
  - Chronic ingestion (i.e., greater than 100 mg/kg/day for more than 2 days) can be more serious than acute ingestion

TREATMENT

- Decrease GI absorption—gastric lavage and activated charcoal.
- Provide oxygen or mechanical ventilation assistance as necessary.
- Treat for hyperthermia (external cool down, tepid water sponge bath), dehydration (IV hydration, balance pH, and electrolytes), bleeding (vitamin K), seizures (anticonvulsants), and reverse acidosis (slow infusion of bicarbonate).
- Hemodialysis or peritoneal dialysis may be required in severe cases.

NURSING IMPLICATIONS

1. Teach parents safe medication storage.
2. Teach parents not to administer aspirin to children who are suspected of having a viral infection, especially chickenpox or influenza.
3. Do not administer aspirin to patients younger than 18 years; Reye syndrome may occur.
4. Monitor respiratory status, blood gases, and the progression of symptoms.
5. Assist older adult patients to evaluate the combination of over-the-counter (OTC) medications for the presence of aspirin.
6. Aspirin overdose needs to be treated at an emergency center.

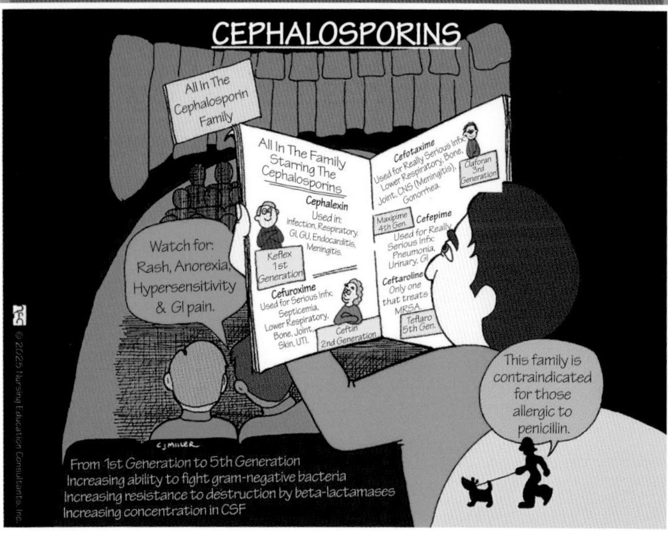
CEPHALOSPORINS
All In The Cephalosporin Family
All In The Family Starring The Cephalosporins
Cephalexin
Used in: Infection, Respiratory, GI, GU, Endocarditis, Meningitis.
Keflex 1st Generation
Cefuroxime
Used for Serious Infx: Septicemia, Lower Respiratory, Bone, Joint, Skin, UTI.
Ceftin 2nd Generation
Cefotaxime
Used for Really Serious Infx: Lower Respiratory, Bone, Joint, CNS (Meningitis), Gonorrhea.
Claforan 3rd Generation
Maxipime 4th Gen.
Cefepime
Used for Really Serious Infx: Pneumonia, Urinary, GI
Ceftaroline
Only one that treats MRSA.
Teflaro 5th Gen.
Watch for: Rash, Anorexia, Hypersensitivity & GI pain.
This family is contraindicated for those allergic to penicillin.
From 1st Generation to 5th Generation
Increasing ability to fight gram-negative bacteria
Increasing resistance to destruction by beta-lactamases
Increasing concentration in CSF
© 2025 Nursing Education Consultants, Inc.

What You Need to Know

Cephalosporins

ACTION

Each generation has increasing bactericidal activity to break down gram-negative bacteria and anaerobes, as well as to reach the cerebrospinal fluid. Cephalosporins interfere with bacterial cell wall synthesis and are considered broad-spectrum antibiotics. The cell weakens, swells, bursts, and dies as a result of increased osmotic pressure inside the cell. Increased cephalosporin resistance is caused by production of beta-lactamases.

USES

- Gram-negative and gram-positive bacterial infections; not active against viral or fungal infections

CAUTION

- Do not use in patients with a severe penicillin allergy (anaphylaxis, hives)

SIDE EFFECTS (VERY SIMILAR TO PENICILLIN)

- Hypersensitivity reactions: rash, pruritus, fever.
- Anorexia, nausea, flatulence, vomiting, diarrhea.
- Can promote a *Clostridium difficile* infection.
- Severe immediate anaphylactic reactions are rare.
- Cefazolin, ceftriaxone, and cefotetan may cause bleeding tendencies.
- Taking cefotetan or cefazolin and drinking alcohol may cause a serious disulfiram-like reaction.

NURSING IMPLICATIONS

1. Evaluate intramuscular (IM) and intravenous (IV) sites for reaction, such as abscess and thrombophlebitis. Minimize complication of thrombophlebitis by rotating injection sites and slowly injecting in a dilute solution.
2. IM injections are frequently painful; forewarn patient.
3. Do not reconstitute ceftriaxone with any calcium diluents (Ringer solution).
4. Notify health care provider (HCP) if diarrhea occurs—can promote development of *C. difficile* infection.
5. Monitor kidney and hepatic studies throughout therapy.
6. With medications that cause bleeding tendencies, monitor for bleeding.
7. If gastrointestinal (GI) upset occurs, patient can take medication with food.
8. Teach patient to refrigerate oral suspensions.
9. Instruct patient to report any signs of allergy (e.g., skin rash, itching, hives).

TETRACYCLINE USES

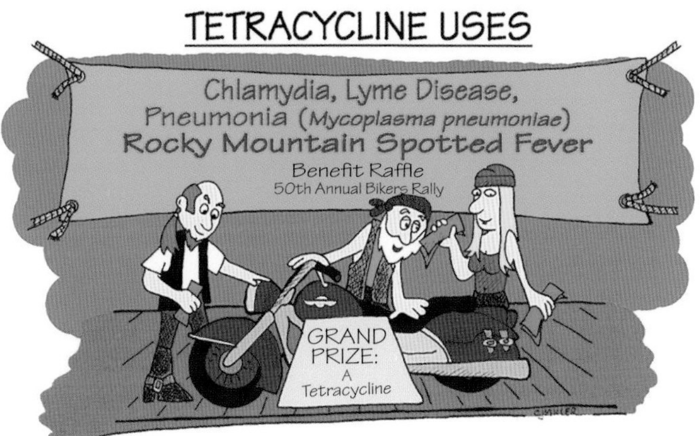

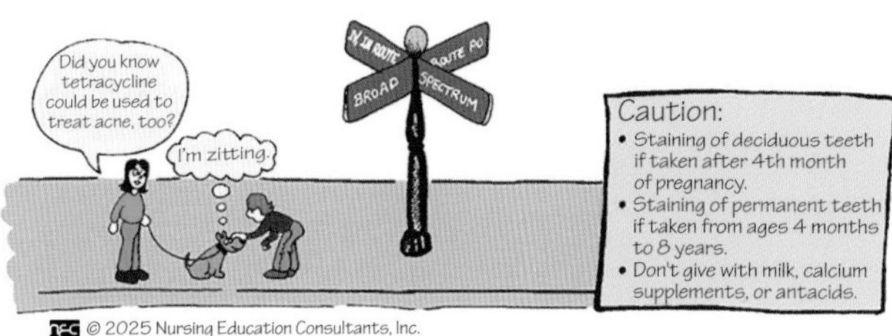

What You Need to Know

Tetracyclines

CLASSIFICATION

Antibiotics

ACTION

Tetracyclines are bacteriostatic, broad-spectrum antibiotics that suppress bacterial growth by inhibiting protein synthesis. Inhibit growth of both gram-negative and gram-positive bacteria.

USES

- Rickettsial diseases (Rocky Mountain spotted fever, typhus, Q fever)
- *Chlamydia* infections, peptic ulcer disease (*Helicobacter pylori* infection)
- Acne, *Mycoplasma pneumoniae*, Lyme disease, periodontal disease
- Brucellosis, cholera, anthrax

PRECAUTIONS

- Tetracycline and demeclocycline should not be given to patients with kidney disease.
- May exacerbate kidney impairment; hepatotoxicity.
- Do not give to children younger than 8 years, pregnant women, or breast-feeding women.
- May cause staining of developing teeth and permanent tooth discoloration.

SIDE EFFECTS

- Alteration of vaginal and intestinal flora resulting in diarrhea and GI upset
- Dizziness, light-headedness, diarrhea, nausea, vomiting, abdominal cramps
- Photosensitivity, superinfection (*C. difficile*)

NURSING IMPLICATIONS

1. Monitor carefully for diarrhea; it may indicate a superinfection of bowel (*C. difficile* or *Staphylococci*).
2. Check dose and rate when delivering IV.
3. Take 1 hour before or 2 hours after ingestion of antacids, milk products, magnesium-containing laxatives, calcium supplements, and iron supplements.
4. To avoid discoloration of teeth, do not administer to pregnant women, breast-feeding women, or children younger than 8 years.
5. Use a straw with liquid preparations.
6. Wear sunscreen and protective clothing.

Important nursing implications	Serious/life-threatening implications
Most frequent side effects	Patient teaching

METRONIDAZOLE (FLAGYL)

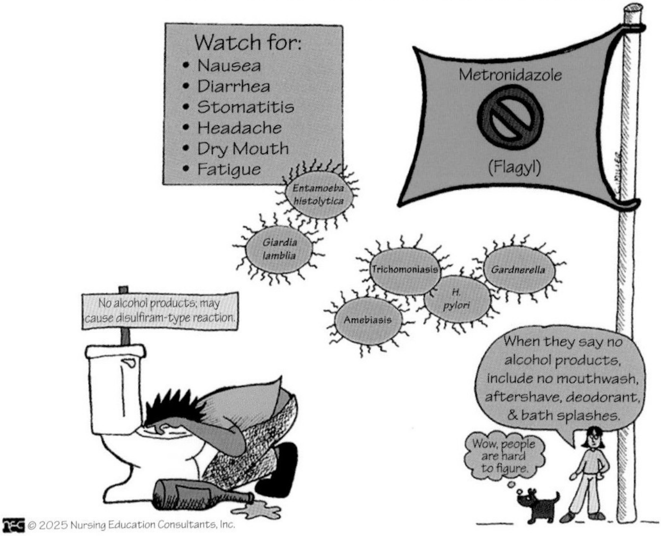

Watch for:
- Nausea
- Diarrhea
- Stomatitis
- Headache
- Dry Mouth
- Fatigue

Metronidazole

(Flagyl)

Entamoeba histolytica

Giardia lamblia

Trichomoniasis

Gardnerella

H. pylori

Amebiasis

No alcohol products; may cause disulfiram-type reaction.

When they say no alcohol products, include no mouthwash, aftershave, deodorant, & bath splashes.

Wow, people are hard to figure.

What You Need to Know

Metronidazole (Flagyl)

CLASSIFICATION

Antibacterial/antiprotozoal

ACTION

Bactericidal effects against anaerobic bacterial pathogens as well as several protozoa. Interacts with cell DNA to cause strand breakage and loss of helical structure. The impairment of DNA is responsible for the antimicrobial and mutagenic actions of the medication.

USES

- Asymptomatic and symptomatic trichomoniasis in female and male patients
- Acute intestinal amebiasis, giardiasis, *C. difficile* infection, antibiotic-associated colitis
- Used in combination with tetracycline and bismuth subsalicylate (Pepto-Bismol) for treatment of *H. pylori*
- Given prophylactically in colorectal, abdominal, gynecologic surgical procedures

PRECAUTIONS

- Active central nervous system (CNS) disease, blood dyscrasias
- Avoid during first-trimester pregnancy, breast-feeding
- Second- and third-trimester pregnancies-use with caution
- Alcoholism, hepatic disease

SIDE EFFECTS

- Nausea, headache, dry mouth, vomiting, diarrhea, vertigo, weakness
- Metallic taste, darkening of the urine, stomatitis, insomnia
- Rarely, seizures, peripheral neuropathy, encephalopathy, aseptic meningitis
- Hypersensitivity reactions, Stevens-Johnson syndrome

NURSING IMPLICATIONS

1. Take on an empty stomach if possible; may take with food if nauseated.
2. Do not use products containing alcohol (cologne, aftershave lotion, or bath splashes) or ingest alcohol products to avoid a disulfiram-type reaction (e.g., flushing, nausea and vomiting, palpitations, tachycardia, psychosis).
3. Wait until 24 hours after last dose of drug to resume breast-feeding.
4. Teach patient that harmless darkening of the urine may occur.

Important nursing implications — Serious/life-threatening implications

Most frequent side effects — Patient teaching

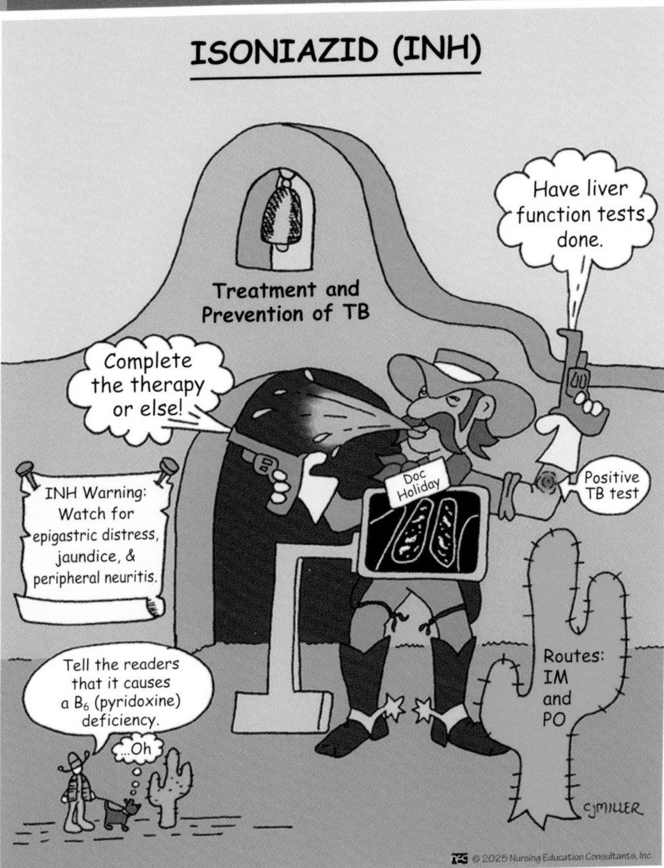
ISONIAZID (INH)
Treatment and Prevention of TB
Have liver function tests done.
Complete the therapy or else!
Doc Holiday
Positive TB test
INH Warning: Watch for epigastric distress, jaundice, & peripheral neuritis.
Tell the readers that it causes a B6 (pyridoxine) deficiency.
...Oh
Routes: IM and PO
CJMILLER
© 2025 Nursing Education Consultants, Inc.

What You Need to Know

Isoniazid

CLASSIFICATION

Antimycobacterial, antituberculosis agent

ACTION ■ Black Box Warning

Causes disruption of bacterial cell wall, loss of acid-fast properties in susceptible mycobacteria. Bactericidal against actively growing intracellular, extracellular susceptible mycobacteria.

USES

- Treatment of active and latent tuberculosis (TB) infection
- Preventive in high-risk persons (e.g., those with a positive TB skin test or exposure)

CONTRAINDICATIONS AND PRECAUTIONS

- History of isoniazid (INH)-associated hypersensitivity reaction.
- Patients with alcoholism or preexisting liver problems.
- Severe, potentially fatal hepatitis may occur.

SIDE EFFECTS

- Dose-related peripheral neuropathy, paresthesia (tingling, numbness, burning, pain), clumsiness, unsteadiness, muscle ache
- Epigastric distress, jaundice, drug-induced hepatitis

NURSING IMPLICATIONS

1. Teach patient to take orally on an empty stomach 1 hour before or 2 hours after meals.
2. Depletes vitamin B_6 (pyridoxine); patient will need supplementation during treatment.
3. Peripheral neuropathy, the most common adverse effect, is preceded by paresthesia (e.g., numbness, tingling, burning, pain) of the feet and hands.
4. Teach patient to reduce or eliminate consumption of alcohol to reduce risk of hepatotoxicity.
5. Treatment always involves two or more medications for active TB; INH is often combined with rifampin.

Remember the mnemonic **STRIPE** for antibiotics used in TB:
ST—**ST**reptomycin; **R**—**R**ifampin; **I**—**I**NH; **P**—**P**yrazinamide; **E**—**E**thambutol

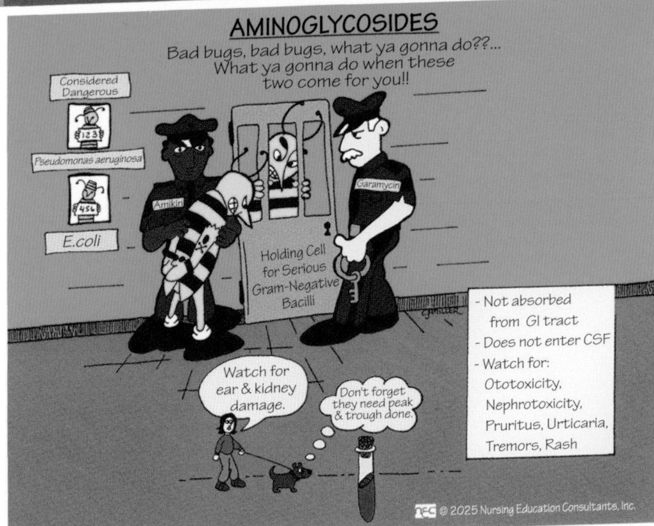
AMINOGLYCOSIDES
Bad bugs, bad bugs, what ya gonna do??...
What ya gonna do when these
two come for you!!
Considered
Dangerous
123
Pseudomonas aeruginosa
456
E.coli
Amikin
Garamycin
Holding Cell
for Serious
Gram-Negative
Bacilli
- Not absorbed
from GI tract
- Does not enter CSF
- Watch for:
Ototoxicity,
Nephrotoxicity,
Pruritus, Urticaria,
Tremors, Rash
Watch for
ear & kidney
damage.
Don't forget
they need peak
& trough done.
© 2025 Nursing Education Consultants, Inc.

What You Need to Know

Aminoglycosides

ACTION ■ Black Box Warning

Primarily effective against bacterial infections caused by aerobic gram-negative bacilli. Disrupts the cell synthesis of protein; cell kill is dependent on the concentration of the medication. The higher the concentration, the more rapidly the infection will clear.

USES

- Parenteral use (poorly absorbed orally) for treatment of serious infections of the GI, respiratory, urinary tracts; CNS; bone; skin and soft tissue, including burns
- Topically for local infection to eyes, ears, skin
- Active TB, tularemia, plague

CONTRAINDICATION

- History of hypersensitivity or toxic reaction with aminoglycoside antibiotics

PRECAUTIONS

- Patients who have kidney impairment
- History of hearing impairment
- Patients with myasthenia gravis
- Possible fetal damage when given to pregnant women

SIDE EFFECTS

- Nephrotoxicity (reversible injury) and ototoxicity (irreversible injury)
- Neuromuscular blockade leading to flaccid paralysis and fatal respiratory depression; increased risk in patients receiving skeletal muscle relaxants
- Hypersensitivity reactions: rash, urticaria, pruritus

NURSING IMPLICATIONS

1. Peak and trough levels should be assessed. Ototoxicity is associated with persistent high trough levels rather than high peak levels.
2. Monitor kidney function (e.g., blood urea nitrogen [BUN], creatinine levels).
3. Monitor for sensory problems (e.g., loss of hearing, balance).
4. Instruct patients to report tinnitus, high-frequency hearing loss, persistent headache, nausea, dizziness, vertigo.
5. Anticipate antidote of IV calcium gluconate for treatment of neuromuscular blockade.
6. Penicillins and aminoglycosides should not be mixed together in the same IV solution because penicillin can inactivate the aminoglycoside.

AMINOGLYCOSIDE TOXICITY

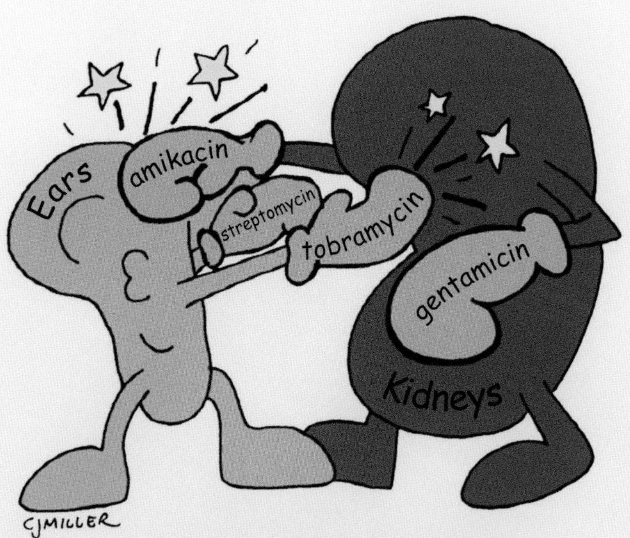

Major toxic effects of aminoglycosides are ototoxicity and nephrotoxicity.

What You Need to Know

Aminoglycoside Toxicity

ACTION (AMINOGLYCOSIDE ANTIBIOTICS) ■ Black Box Warning

Bactericidal against gram-negative bacteria and certain gram-positive organisms. Disrupts bacterial protein synthesis. Used for serious infections.

CONTRAINDICATIONS AND PRECAUTIONS

- History of hypersensitivity or toxic reaction with aminoglycoside antibiotics
- Patients with kidney impairment, history of hearing impairment
- Concurrent use with nephrotoxic drugs (amphotericin B, cephalosporins, vancomycin, cyclosporine, aspirin, nonsteroidal anti-inflammatory drugs [NSAIDs])
- Patients with myasthenia gravis
- Older adults

TOXICITY

- Nephrotoxicity (reversible injury) and ototoxicity (irreversible injury).
- Neuromuscular blockade can lead to flaccid paralysis, and fatal respiratory depression can occur in patients receiving skeletal muscle relaxants.

DRUG INTERACTIONS

- Loop diuretics, specifically ethacrynic acid (Edecrin), significantly increases ototoxicity.
- Amphotericin B, cephalosporins, polymyxins, vancomycin, cyclosporine, acetylsalicylic acid, and NSAIDs increase risk of nephrotoxicity.
- Skeletal muscle relaxants and neuromuscular-blocking agents used in surgery increase risk of neuromuscular blockade.

NURSING IMPLICATIONS

1. Peak and trough levels should be assessed. Ototoxicity is associated with persistent high trough levels rather than high peak levels.
2. Monitor kidney function (e.g., BUN, creatinine levels).
3. Monitor for sensory problems (e.g., loss of hearing, balance).
4. Instruct patients to report tinnitus, high-frequency hearing loss, persistent headache, nausea, dizziness, vertigo.
5. Anticipate antidote of IV calcium gluconate for treatment of neuromuscular blockade.

Important nursing implications | Serious/life-threatening implications

Most frequent side effects | Patient teaching

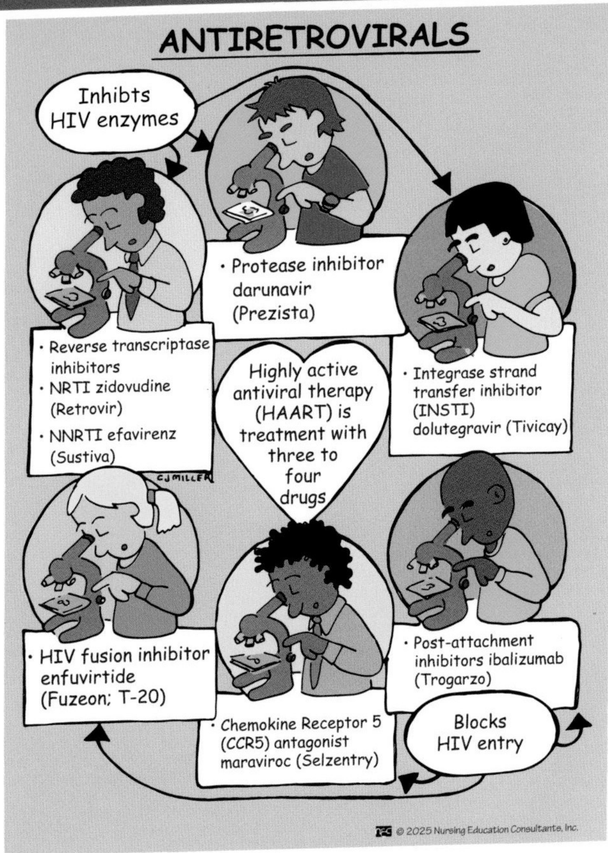
ANTIRETROVIRALS
Inhibts HIV enzymes
• Protease inhibitor darunavir (Prezista)
• Reverse transcriptase inhibitors
• NRTI zidovudine (Retrovir)
• NNRTI efavirenz (Sustiva)
• Integrase strand transfer inhibitor (INSTI) dolutegravir (Tivicay)
Highly active antiviral therapy (HAART) is treatment with three to four drugs
CJMILLER
• HIV fusion inhibitor enfuvirtide (Fuzeon; T-20)
• Post-attachment inhibitors ibalizumab (Trogarzo)
• Chemokine Receptor 5 (CCR5) antagonist maraviroc (Selzentry)
Blocks HIV entry
© 2025 Nursing Education Consultants, Inc.

What You Need to Know

Antiretrovirals

ACTIONS ■ Black Box Warning

- Nucleoside/nucleotide reverse transcriptase inhibitors (NRTIs), nonnucleoside reverse transcriptase inhibitors (NNRTIs), protease inhibitors (PIs), integrase strand transfer inhibitors (INSTIs)—inhibit enzymes required for human immunodeficiency virus (HIV) replication
- HIV fusion inhibitors, postattachment inhibitors, and chemokine receptor 5 (CCR5) antagonists—block entry of virus into CD4-T cells

CONTRAINDICATIONS AND PRECAUTIONS

- Known hypersensitivity and/or intolerable toxicity

SIDE EFFECTS

- *NRTI:* anemia and neutropenia from bone marrow suppression, GI upset; rarely lactic acidosis and hepatic steatosis (fatty liver)
- *NNRTI:* CNS symptoms (dizziness, insomnia, drowsiness); rash may range from mild to severe; check liver function studies
- *PI:* hyperglycemia, fat maldistribution (pseudo-Cushing syndrome), hyperlipidemia, bone loss, elevation in serum transaminases (liver injury)
- *HIV fusion inhibitor:* injection site reactions, pneumonia, hypersensitivity
- *CCR5 antagonist:* cough, dizziness, pyrexia, rash, abdominal pain
- *INSTI:* Stevens-Johnson syndrome, toxic epidermal necrolysis
- *Postattachment inhibitors:* infusion reactions, hypersensitivity

NURSING IMPLICATIONS

1. Check to see whether medication should be taken with or without food because this varies with drug classes.
2. Instruct patient to take the full dose and complete treatment regimen.
3. Pregnant women should receive antiretroviral therapy regardless of pregnancy status.
4. Teach patient to report symptoms related to severe rash, CNS issues, elevated blood glucose, pneumonia.
5. Monitor CD4-T-cell count—medications do not cure or kill HIV, but slow down replication.

Remember, **vir** at the start, middle, or end of a word means virus: acyclo**vir**, efa**vir**enz, enfu**vir**tide, retro**vir**, saquina**vir** (In**vir**ase), mara**vir**oc.

PRE-EXPOSURE PROPHYLAXIS (PrEP)

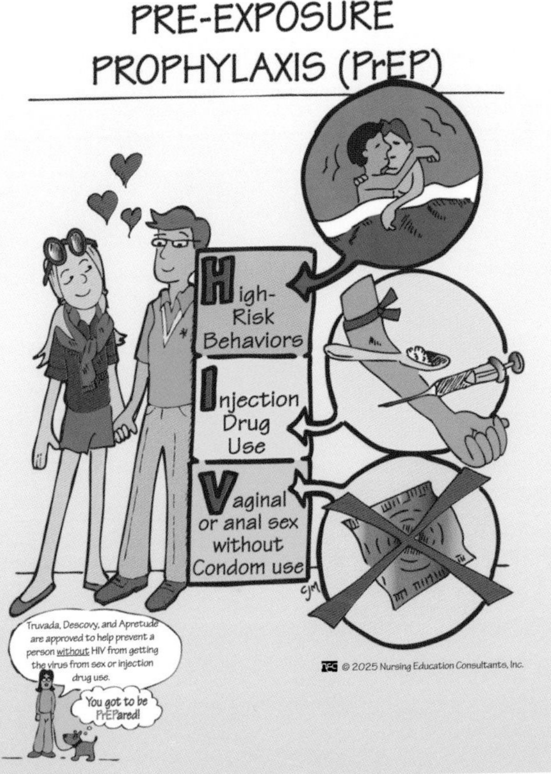

What You Need to Know

Pre-Exposure Prophylaxis

Pre-exposure prophylaxis (PrEP) is when people at risk for HIV take medicine to prevent HIV. PrEP is highly effective for preventing HIV from sex or injection drug use. Three antiretroviral medications are approved:

- Emtricitabine and tenofovir disoproxil fumarate (Truvada)—recommended to prevent HIV for all people at risk through sex or injection drug use
- Emtricitabine and tenofovir alafenamide (Descovy)—recommended to prevent HIV for people at risk through sex, excluding people at risk through receptive vaginal sex
- Cabotegravir (Apretude)—long-acting injectable given to protect against HIV in adults and adolescents who weigh at least 77 lb

ACTIONS ■ Black Box Warning

- Interferes with HIV viral replication

CONTRAINDICATIONS AND PRECAUTIONS

- Severe liver problems have been known to occur.
- Medication can worsen hepatitis B virus infection with Truvada.
- Sometimes fatal lactic acidosis can occur.
- Contraindicated with patients in kidney failure.
- Apretude may cause mood changes, depression, suicidal ideation.

SIDE EFFECTS

- Truvada: headache, abdominal pain, weight loss
- Descovy: diarrhea, nausea, headache, fatigue, abdominal pain
- Apretude: pain at injection site, diarrhea, headache, vomiting, abdominal pain

NURSING IMPLICATIONS

1. Patient must be HIV-negative before starting PrEP.
2. Truvada and Descovy are pills that must be taken daily to be effective.
3. Apretude is an injection given every other month by an HCP after initiation injections have been given 1 month apart for 2 consecutive months.
4. Instruct patient to have follow-up testing at least every 3 months while taking PrEP.
5. Teach patient that if they test positive for HIV-1, they need to contact their HCP immediately, as they will need more medicine than PrEP alone to treat HIV.

Important nursing implications | Serious/life-threatening implications
Most frequent side effects | Patient teaching

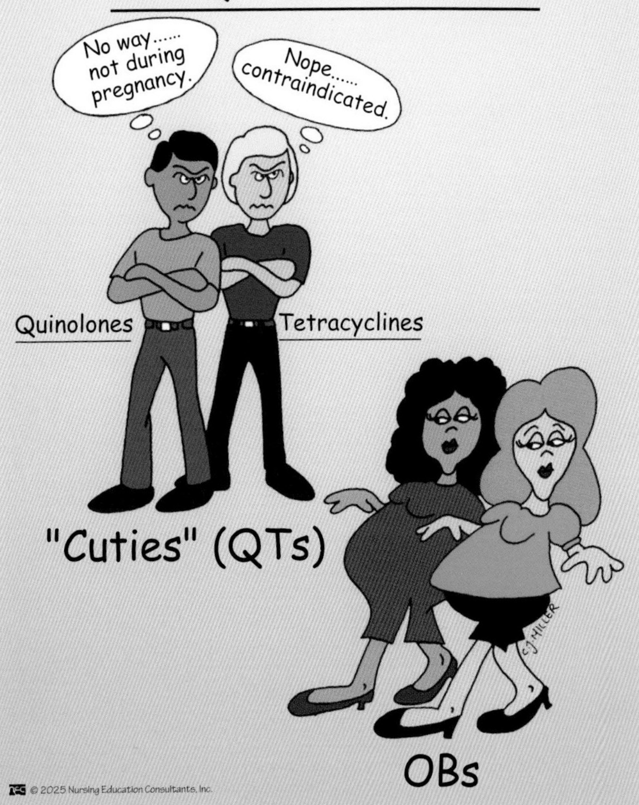
TWO QTs SAY NO TO OBs
No way...... not during pregnancy.
Nope...... contraindicated.
Quinolones
Tetracyclines
"Cuties" (QTs)
OBs
C.J. MILLER
© 2025 Nursing Education Consultants, Inc.

What You Need to Know

Quinolones and Tetracyclines—Drug Impact on Pregnancies

FOOD AND DRUG ADMINISTRATION PREGNANCY AND LACTATIONS LABELING RULE (PLLR) ■ Black Box Warning

- The PLLR requires three sections for labeling: (1) pregnancy, (2) lactation, and (3) females and males of reproductive potential. These are further divided into subsections containing specified content.

CONTRAINDICATIONS

- Women who are pregnant need to take a cautious approach to drug therapy during pregnancy. The HCP is responsible for ordering medications that are safe and appropriate for the ever-changing physiologic dynamics during pregnancy.
- Contraindicated medications can cause detrimental changes in the mother, fetus, and fetal environment.
- Quinolones and tetracyclines are not routinely used during pregnancy.

NURSING IMPLICATIONS

1. Evaluate patient's level of understanding about her physiologic, mental, and emotional conditions.
2. Teach patient to call the prenatal clinic or physician's office before using any over-the-counter medications.
3. The patient should not take any medications that have not been specifically approved or prescribed by her HCP.
4. Advise patient to avoid all alcoholic beverages during the pregnancy term.
5. Advise patient to report any unusual signs or symptoms of reactions to the treatment plan.

Think of the mnemonic **MCAT** to remember other antibiotics contraindicated in pregnancy. **M**—**M**etronidazole; **C**—**C**hloramphenicol; **A**—**A**minoglycoside: **T**—**T**etracycline

Important nursing implications | Serious/life-threatening implications
Most frequent side effects | Patient teaching

FLUOROQUINOLONES

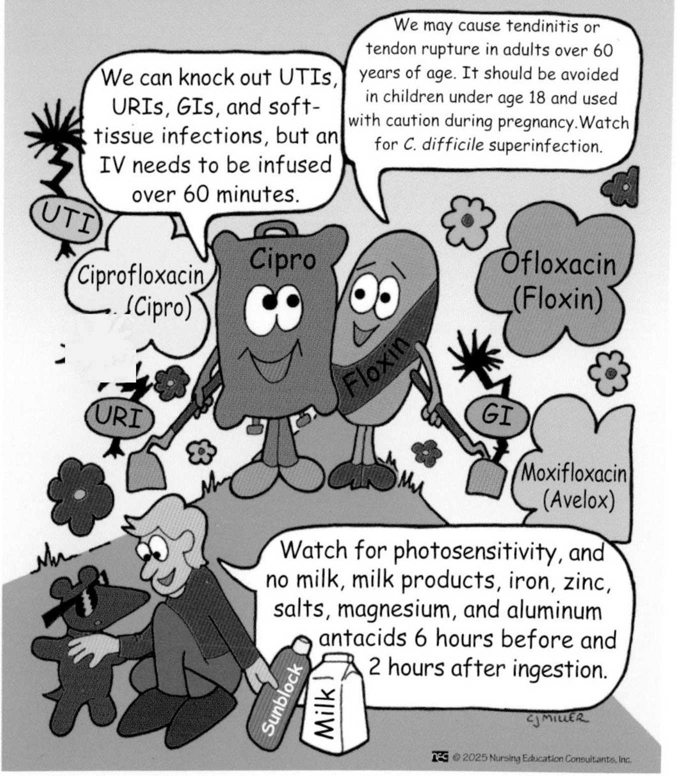

We can knock out UTIs, URIs, GIs, and soft-tissue infections, but an IV needs to be infused over 60 minutes.

We may cause tendinitis or tendon rupture in adults over 60 years of age. It should be avoided in children under age 18 and used with caution during pregnancy. Watch for *C. difficile* superinfection.

UTI

Ciprofloxacin (Cipro)

Cipro

Floxin

Ofloxacin (Floxin)

URI

GI

Moxifloxacin (Avelox)

Watch for photosensitivity, and no milk, milk products, iron, zinc, salts, magnesium, and aluminum antacids 6 hours before and 2 hours after ingestion.

Sunblock

Milk

CJ MILLER

What You Need to Know

Fluoroquinolones

CLASSIFICATION

Antibacterial

ACTIONS ■ Black Box Warning

Bactericidal; inhibits DNA enzyme that interferes with replication; is considered a broad-spectrum antibiotic against most gram-negative and some gram-positive bacteria, but not against anaerobic infections.

USES

- Respiratory, urinary, GI, bone, joint, skin, soft-tissue infections
- Preferred drug for treatment of inhaled anthrax

CONTRAINDICATIONS AND PRECAUTIONS

- Hypersensitivity, history of myasthenia gravis
- Children younger than 18 years (systemic treatment should be avoided)
- Pregnancy

SIDE EFFECTS

- GI upset—nausea, vomiting, diarrhea, abdominal pain
- Dizziness, headache, restlessness
- Patients older than 60 years, patients taking glucocorticoids, and patients who have undergone a heart, liver, or kidney transplantation are at highest risk for tendinitis and tendon rupture
- Photosensitivity reactions: patients should avoid sunlight and sunlamps
- Avoid moxifloxacin in patients with prolonged QT interval, hypokalemia, those taking prodysrhythmic drugs
- Older adults—confusion, visual disturbances, somnolence, psychosis
- *C. difficile* infection

NURSING IMPLICATIONS

1. Teach patient to avoid antacids, calcium supplements, iron supplements, dairy products, and aluminum- or magnesium-containing antacids for at least 6 hours before and 2 hours after taking medication; encourage adequate fluid intake.
2. Teach patient to report any tendon pain or inflammation.
3. Ciprofloxacin and ofloxacin can increase theophylline levels and warfarin levels—monitor theophylline levels and prothrombin time in patients taking theophylline or warfarin.
4. Monitor for prolonged QT interval in patients with cardiac disease taking antidysrhythmic agents.
5. Teach patient to wear sunscreen and protective clothing when in sunlight.

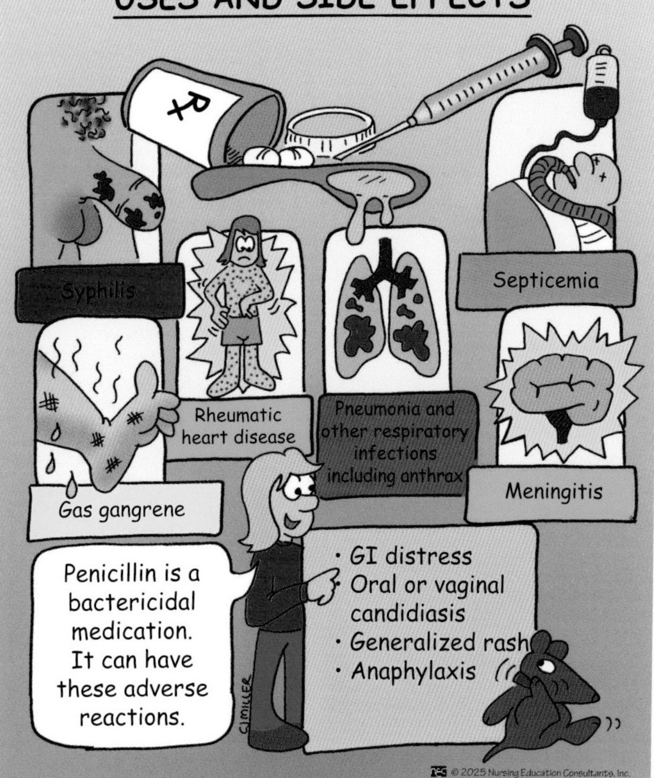
PENICILLIN (PCN)
USES AND SIDE EFFECTS
Syphilis
Septicemia
Rheumatic heart disease
Pneumonia and other respiratory infections including anthrax
Meningitis
Gas gangrene
Penicillin is a bactericidal medication. It can have these adverse reactions.
· GI distress
· Oral or vaginal candidiasis
· Generalized rash
· Anaphylaxis
CJ MILLER
© 2025 Nursing Education Consultants, Inc.

What You Need to Know

Penicillin

ACTION

Bactericidal; disrupts and weakens the cell wall, leading to cell lysis and death.

USE

- Treatment of bacterial infections based on type of penicillin

TYPES

- Narrow-spectrum penicillinase-*sensitive*—penicillin G (Bicillin), penicillin V
- Narrow-spectrum penicillinase-*resistant* (antistaphylococcal penicillins)—nafcillin, oxacillin, dicloxacillin
- Broad-spectrum (aminopenicillins)—ampicillin, amoxicillin, amoxicillin/clavulanate (Augmentin)
- Extended-spectrum penicillins (antipseudomonal penicillins)—piperacillin/tazobactam (Zosyn)

CONTRAINDICATIONS AND PRECAUTIONS

- Hypersensitivity or any history of allergic reaction to penicillin
- Caution in patients with allergy to cephalosporin, depending on severity of allergic response

SIDE EFFECTS

- Allergic response (all types)—rash, itching, hives, anaphylaxis.
- High IV doses of sodium penicillin G can produce sodium overload. Exercise caution in patients under sodium restriction (e.g., patients with cardiac disease, hypertension).

NURSING IMPLICATIONS

1. Instruct patient to check label with regard to administering with food.
2. Instruct patient to wear medication-alert bracelet if allergic to penicillin.
3. Monitor kidney and cardiac function and electrolyte levels to avoid untoward effects.
4. Monitor patient for 30 minutes when given parenterally; administer epinephrine if anaphylaxis occurs.
5. Collect any laboratory culture specimens before initiating penicillin therapy.
6. Do not mix aminoglycosides with penicillin in the same IV infusion—deactivates the aminoglycoside.
7. When administering parenterally, be careful to avoid intra-arterial injection or injection into peripheral nerves because serious injury can result.

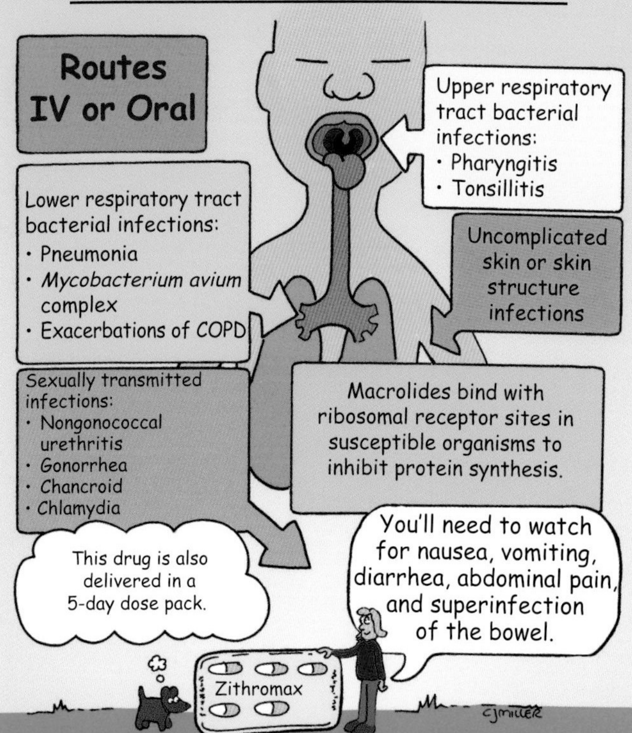
MACROLIDES
Top to Bottom...Mild to Moderate
Routes
IV or Oral
Upper respiratory tract bacterial infections:
• Pharyngitis
• Tonsillitis
Lower respiratory tract bacterial infections:
• Pneumonia
• Mycobacterium avium complex
• Exacerbations of COPD
Uncomplicated skin or skin structure infections
Sexually transmitted infections:
• Nongonococcal urethritis
• Gonorrhea
• Chancroid
• Chlamydia
Macrolides bind with ribosomal receptor sites in susceptible organisms to inhibit protein synthesis.
This drug is also delivered in a 5-day dose pack.
You'll need to watch for nausea, vomiting, diarrhea, abdominal pain, and superinfection of the bowel.
Zithromax
CJMILLER
© 2025 Nursing Education Consultants, Inc.

What You Need to Know

Macrolides

ACTION

Broad-spectrum antibiotic that binds with ribosomal receptor sites in susceptible organisms to inhibit bacterial protein synthesis.

USES

- There are three main drugs:
  - Erythromycin—drug of choice for *Bordetella pertussis* (whooping cough), acute diphtheria
  - Azithromycin—drug of choice for *Chlamydia trachomatis*
  - Clarithromycin—treats *Mycobacterium avium* complex
- Treats upper respiratory tract, ear, skin infections; syphilis (for penicillin-sensitive patients); cholera; chancroid
- Used as a substitute for penicillin G in penicillin-allergic patients

CONTRAINDICATIONS AND PRECAUTIONS

- Liver dysfunction
- Avoid macrolides in patients with preexisting QT prolongation and in those taking drugs that can increase erythromycin levels (e.g., verapamil, diltiazem, HIV PIs, azole antifungal drugs).
- Patients taking theophylline, warfarin, digoxin, carbamazepine, or tacrolimus—monitor closely for signs of toxicity.

SIDE EFFECTS

- Diarrhea, nausea and vomiting, abdominal pain.
- High levels of all forms of erythromycin can prolong the QT interval, thereby posing a risk of potentially fatal cardiac dysrhythmias.

NURSING IMPLICATIONS

1. Take medication 1 hour before or 2 hours after food or antacids.
2. Aluminum and magnesium antacids reduce rate of absorption but not extent.
3. Observe for development of signs of superinfection.
4. Instruct patient to take prescribed course of therapy, although symptoms may improve or disappear.
5. IV preparations are infused slowly over 60 minutes.

THE AZOLES

"One Way to Say No to Fungus!"

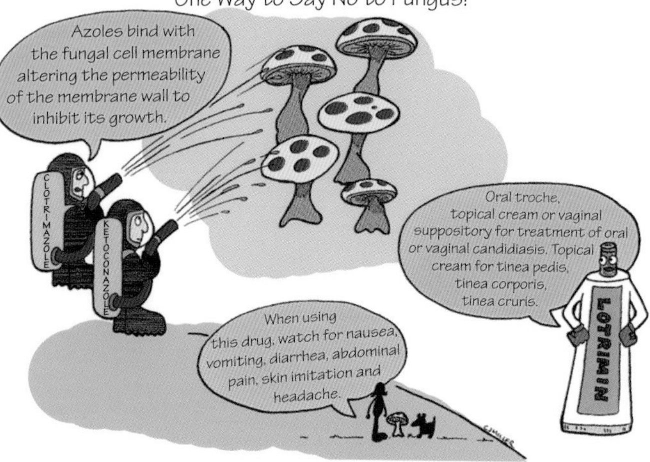

What You Need to Know

The Azoles

CLASSIFICATION

Antifungal

ACTION

Broad-spectrum antifungal that inhibits an essential component of the fungal cytoplasmic membrane.

USES

- Superficial mycoses caused by *Candida* species and dermatophytes (species of *Epidermophyton*, *Trichophyton*, *Microsporum*).
- *Candida* infections usually occur in mucous membranes and moist skin; chronic infections may involve the scalp, skin, and nails.
- Dermatophytoses are generally confined to the skin, hair, and nails.

CONTRAINDICATIONS AND PRECAUTIONS

- Precaution with pregnancy
- Chronic liver disease

SIDE EFFECTS

- Topical application: stinging, erythema, edema, urticaria, pruritus, peeling.
- Intravaginal administration may cause a burning sensation and abdominal cramping.
- Oral therapy (clotrimazole) can cause GI distress.

NURSING IMPLICATIONS

1. Administer oral tablets 2 hours prior to antacids to prevent decreased absorption due to the high pH of gastric contents.
2. Teach that condoms and diaphragms may be weakened if they are used during treatment with vaginal clotrimazole.
3. Teach patient to call their HCP if they still have symptoms of infection 7 days after starting treatment with clotrimazole.
4. Teach patient to avoid intercourse while using a vaginal preparation.

Important nursing implications | Serious/life-threatening implications
Most frequent side effects | Patient teaching

MUPIROCIN TOPICAL ANTIBIOTIC

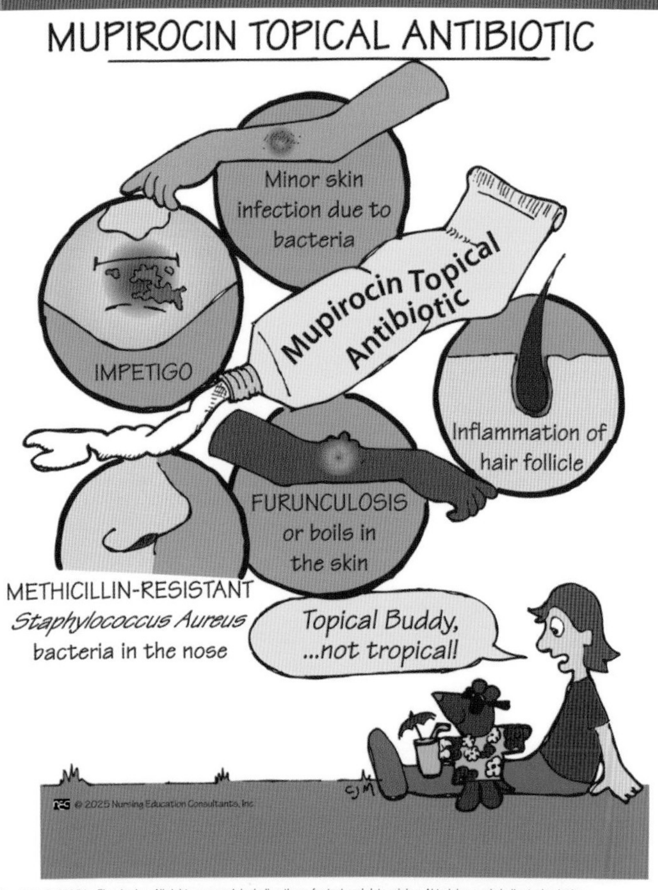

What You Need to Know

Mupirocin

ACTION

Topical antibiotic that blocks protein synthesis and is bactericidal at therapeutic concentrations.

USES

- Treatment of impetigo caused by *Staphylococcus aureus*, *Streptococcus pyogenes*, or beta-hemolytic *Streptococcus*
- Elimination of nasal colonization caused by methicillin-resistant *S. aureus*
- Folliculitis, furunculosis (boils)

CONTRAINDICATIONS AND PRECAUTIONS

- Systemic toxicity does not occur owing to minimal absorption from topical sites
- Moderate or severe kidney impairment

SIDE EFFECTS

- Topical: local skin irritation
- Intranasal: headache, rhinitis, upper respiratory congestion, pharyngitis

NURSING IMPLICATIONS

1. Mupirocin is available only in topical formulations—ointment, cream.
2. Apply topical medication after cleansing the area with soap and water, dry well before applying a thin film of the ointment or cream.
3. Intranasal application: apply approximately half of the ointment from the single-use tube directly from the tube into one nostril, then apply the remainder of the ointment directly into the other nostril. Have patient close the nostrils by pressing the sides of the nose together and then releasing them. Do this over and over again for approximately 1 minute; may also press the sides of the nose together and gently massage the nose. This will help spread the medicine throughout the inside of the nostrils. Throw away the single-use tube after application.
4. Do not apply mupirocin to the eyes; it is not for ophthalmic use.
5. Teach patient to continue to use the medication for the full time prescribed, even if symptoms or the skin lesion disappears after a few days. Explain the importance of not stopping the medication too early, because it may result in a return of the infection.

HEPARIN

The Clotting Roundup

I interfere with the activation of fibrin and fibrinogen from thrombin that keeps the clots from forming... Whoa...!

Thrombin

I cannot help you!

Steps to Clotting

Fibrin

Heparin

Heparin prevents fibrin from forming a clot and helps prevent deep vein thrombosis and pulmonary emboli. It doesn't break up a clot; it just keeps it from coming together.

HEPARIN

- Rapid acting
- Given intravenously or subcutaneously
- Need to check activated partial thromboplastin time (aPTT)
- Need bleeding precautions

EJMILLER

What You Need to Know

Heparin

ACTION ▲ High Alert

Heparin is an anticoagulant that exerts a direct effect on blood coagulation by enhancing the inhibitory actions of antithrombin on several factors essential to normal blood clotting, thereby blocking the conversion of prothrombin to thrombin and fibrinogen to fibrin.

USES

- Rapid acting (within minutes) to prevent and treat deep vein thrombosis (DVT), pulmonary embolism (PE), and emboli in atrial fibrillation
- Used to treat disseminated intravascular coagulation
- Is a preferred anticoagulant during pregnancy (does not cross the placenta or enter breast milk)
- Prevents coagulation in heart-lung machines and dialyzers in patients after open-heart surgery and dialysis
- Used as an adjunct to thrombolytic therapy of acute myocardial infarction (MI)

PRECAUTIONS AND CONTRAINDICATIONS

- Bleeding tendencies—hemophilia, dissecting aneurysm, peptic ulcer
- Thrombocytopenia, uncontrollable bleeding, threatened abortion
- Postoperative patients—especially eye, brain, spinal cord surgeries; lumbar puncture; regional anesthesia

SIDE EFFECTS

- Injection site reactions and heparin-induced thrombocytopenia (HIT) may develop
- May result in spontaneous bleeding

NURSING IMPLICATIONS

1. Monitor activated partial thromboplastin time (aPTT)—should be 1½ to 2 times the control value (30-40 seconds) making the aPTT 60 to 70 seconds; anti-Xa assay levels may be used for guiding intravenous (IV) heparin titration; anti-Xa levels of 0.3 to 0.7 IU/mL are considered therapeutic for anticoagulation. Report aPTT >70 seconds to HCP (spontaneous bleeding can occur).
2. *Watch for bleeding*—bruising, petechiae, hypotension, hemoptysis
3. May not be given orally or by intramuscular (IM) injection; protamine sulfate is the antidote.
4. Caution patients not to take aspirin or any medication that decreases platelet aggregation (clopidogrel) unless ordered specifically by health care provider (HCP).
5. Administered either IV or subcutaneously (SubQ); apply firm pressure for 1 to 2 minutes; do not massage the site after injection.
6. Do not inject SubQ within 2 inches of the umbilicus or any scar tissue.
7. Dosage is prescribed in units, not milligrams.

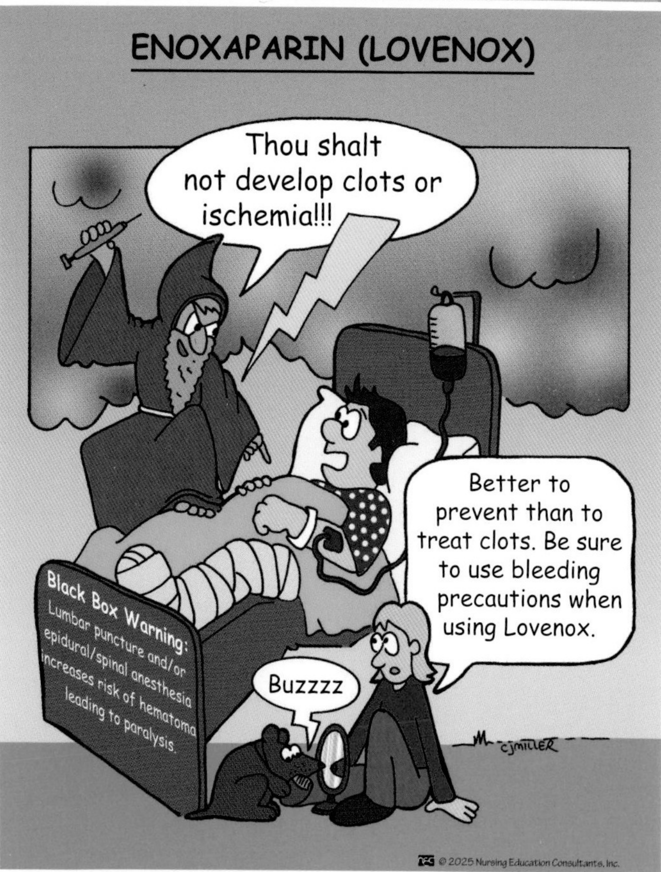
ENOXAPARIN (LOVENOX)
Thou shalt not develop clots or ischemia!!!
Better to prevent than to treat clots. Be sure to use bleeding precautions when using Lovenox.
Black Box Warning: Lumbar puncture and/or epidural/spinal anesthesia increases risk of hematoma leading to paralysis.
Buzzzz
CJMILLER
© 2025 Nursing Education Consultants, Inc.

What You Need to Know

Enoxaparin (Lovenox)

ACTIONS ■ Black Box Warning ▲ High Alert

Low-molecular-weight heparin with a great affinity for factor Xa in providing anticoagulation action; provides a predictable anticoagulant response.

USES

- Prevention of postoperative DVT, pulmonary embolus (PE) PE; prevention of ischemic complications in unstable angina, or non-Q-wave MI, and ST-elevation MI (STEMI); treatment of DVT with or without PE

CONTRAINDICATIONS

- Presence of any active bleeding
- Increased risk of neurologic impairment (permanent paralysis) in patients receiving spinal or epidural anesthesia or undergoing spinal puncture
- Use with caution with concurrent use of aspirin, clopidogrel, other antiplatelet medications
- Not to be used in presence of thrombocytopenia

SIDE EFFECTS

- Immune-mediated thrombocytopenia
- Bleeding episodes

NURSING IMPLICATIONS

1. Medication is only administered SubQ.
2. Protamine sulfate is the antidote.
3. Always double-check—cannot be given to a patient receiving heparin.
4. Injections in abdomen should be 2 inches from the umbilicus or any incisional area.
5. Advise patient not to take any over-the-counter medications, especially aspirin.
6. Check complete blood count (CBC), especially platelet count.
7. Monitor for bleeding:
   - Guaiac stools for occult blood
   - Hematuria
   - Bleeding gums
   - Excessive bruising
8. Does not require aPTT monitoring.

Important nursing implications | Serious/life-threatening implications

Most frequent side effects | Patient teaching

WARFARIN SODIUM (COUMADIN)

Hey Mr. Coumadin, can vitamin K come to our house? We can't make clots without him.

Watch the PT and INR.

101 Liver Road

Clotting Factors

PT

IX

VII

X

As long as I'm in the system, vitamin K won't be able to play.

Coumadin

Vit K

CJMILLER

An overdose of Coumadin can cause hemorrhage, headache, bruising, back pain, ↑ pulse, and ↓ BP.

Coumadin is used to prevent clot formation with DVT, PE, atrial fibrillation, TIA, and coronary occlusive problems.

What You Need to Know

Warfarin Sodium (Coumadin)

ACTIONS ■ Black Box Warning ▲ High Alert

Warfarin is an oral anticoagulant that antagonizes vitamin K, which is necessary for the synthesis of clotting factors VII, IX, X, and prothrombin. As a result, it disrupts the coagulation cascade.

USES

- Long-term prophylaxis of thrombosis; is not useful in an emergency because of delayed onset of action
- Prevents venous thrombosis and thromboembolism associated with atrial fibrillation and prosthetic heart valves
- Decreases risk of recurrent transient ischemic attacks and recurrent MI

CONTRAINDICATIONS

- Bleeding disorders (hemophilia, thrombocytopenia)
- Lumbar puncture; regional anesthesia; or surgery of the eye, brain, or spinal cord
- Vitamin K deficiency; severe hypertension
- Pregnancy and lactation (crosses into breast milk); fetal hemorrhage
- Liver disease, alcoholism

SIDE EFFECTS

- Spontaneous bleeding
- Hypersensitivity reactions (e.g., dermatitis, fever, pruritus, urticaria)
- Red-orange discoloration of urine (not to be confused with hematuria); weakening of bones with long-term use leading to risk of fractures

NURSING IMPLICATIONS

1. Monitor prothrombin time and international normalized ratio (INR) as ordered (2–3 is usually an acceptable INR for anticoagulation).
2. Interacts with a large number of medications; consequently, evaluate medications for interactions before initiating therapy.
3. Monitor for bleeding tendencies; vitamin K (phytonadione) is an antidote.
4. Teach patient to maintain intake of vitamin K (keep constant intake of foods such as green leafy vegetables, mayonnaise, canola oil) and do not abruptly increase or decrease intake.
5. Patient must notify all HCPs that they are taking warfarin, because it is very slow to be excreted from the body.
6. Teach patient to wear a medical alert bracelet.

EPOETIN ALFA (PROCRIT)

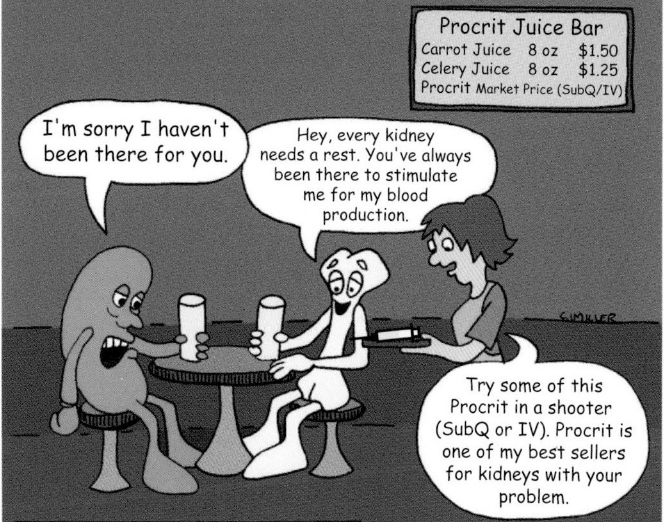

Procrit Juice Bar
Carrot Juice 8 oz $1.50
Celery Juice 8 oz $1.25
Procrit Market Price (SubQ/IV)

I'm sorry I haven't been there for you.

Hey, every kidney needs a rest. You've always been there to stimulate me for my blood production.

Try some of this Procrit in a shooter (SubQ or IV). Procrit is one of my best sellers for kidneys with your problem.

- Procrit is synthetic erythropoietin, which increases RBCs.
- Used to treat anemia associated with kidney failure and chemotherapy.
- Watch for hypertension, headache, and nausea.

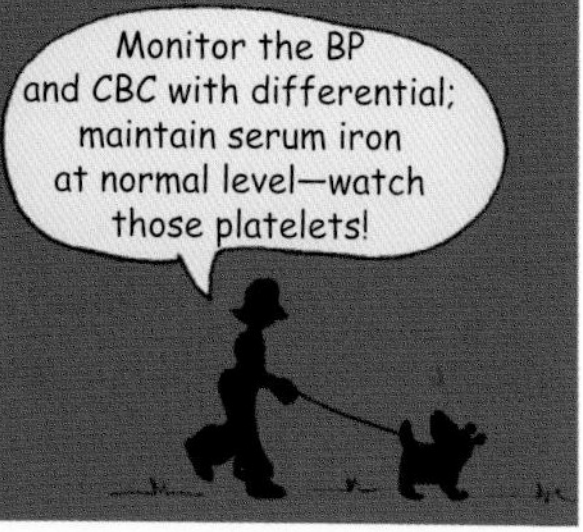

Monitor the BP and CBC with differential; maintain serum iron at normal level—watch those platelets!

What You Need to Know

Epoetin Alfa (Procrit)

ACTION ■ Black Box Warning

Erythropoietic growth factor that stimulates red blood cell (RBC) production in the bone marrow.

USES

- Patients with anemia because of chronic kidney disease, chemotherapy-induced anemia with nonmyeloid malignancies
- Patients infected with human immunodeficiency virus and taking zidovudine (Retrovir)
- Patients with anemia before elective surgery

CONTRAINDICATIONS

- Hemoglobin in excess of 11 gm/dL; hypersensitivity to albumin
- Patients with leukemia or malignant cancers of myeloid origin

PRECAUTIONS

- Poorly controlled hypertension; hypersensitivity to albumin

SIDE EFFECTS

- Hypertension
- Cardiovascular events—cardiac arrest, heart failure, thrombotic events (stroke, MI)
- Patients with cancer—tumor progression and shortened survival
- Autoimmune pure red cell aplasia—severe anemia, RBC production ceases (rarely occurs)

NURSING IMPLICATIONS

1. Monitor blood pressure before erythropoietin therapy.
2. Do not shake solution; it may denature the glycoprotein. Do not mix with other medications.
3. Discard remaining contents because erythropoietin does not contain a preservative.
4. Monitor hemoglobin (Hgb) and hematocrit (Hct), CBC, BUN, creatinine, and serum iron levels as well as fluid and electrolyte balance.
5. Monitor for seizures (rapid increase in Hct level increases risk of hypertensive encephalopathy).
6. Provide patient with required *Medication Guide* from the Food and Drug Administration.

THROMBOLYTICS

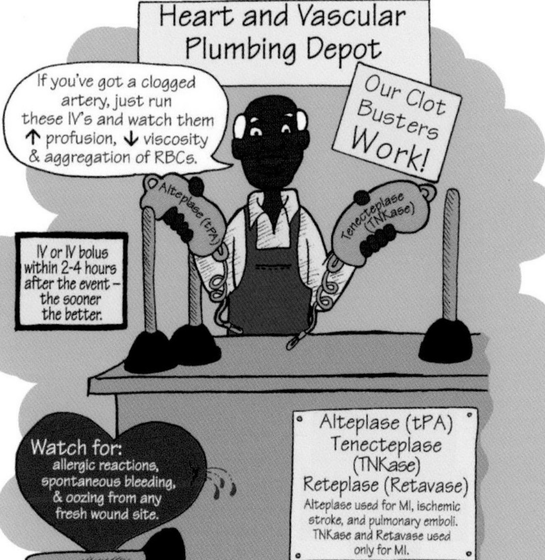

What You Need to Know

Thrombolytics

ACTIONS ▲ High Alert

Work to directly or indirectly convert plasminogen to plasmin, an enzyme that acts to digest the fibrin matrix of clots. Dissolve existing thrombi rather than preventing them from occurring. Also known as *fibrinolytics* or informally as *clot busters*—alteplase (tissue plasminogen activator [tPA]), tenecteplase (TNKase), reteplase (Retavase).

USES

- All three medications used in treatment of acute MI
- tPA used also for PE, acute ischemic stroke, restoring patency in a clogged central venous catheter

CONTRAINDICATIONS AND PRECAUTIONS

- Cerebrovascular disease and pregnancy
- Active internal bleeding, aortic dissection, history of poorly controlled hypertension
- Any prior intracranial hemorrhage or recent head injury
- Recent major surgery or trauma within the prior 2 to 4 weeks
- History of gastrointestinal (GI) bleeding
- Ischemic stroke within past 3 months; except ischemic stroke within 4.5 hours
- Intracranial neoplasm

SIDE EFFECTS

- Hemorrhage (intracranial of greatest concern) and anemia
- Bleeding from recent wounds and needle punctures
- Hypersensitivity reactions—itching, urticaria, headache
- Hypotension, cardiac dysrhythmias

NURSING IMPLICATIONS

1. Administer IV immediately after the event for better outcome, preferably within 2 to 4 hours.
2. Monitor intake and output and Hct levels during treatment.
3. Monitor patient for bleeding and hypersensitivity reactions.
4. While receiving the medication, maintain patient on bed rest; avoid SubQ and IM injections.

Important nursing implications	Serious/life-threatening implications
Most frequent side effects	Patient teaching

CLOPIDOGREL (PLAVIX)

"When platelets gather together, use Plavix for crowd control."

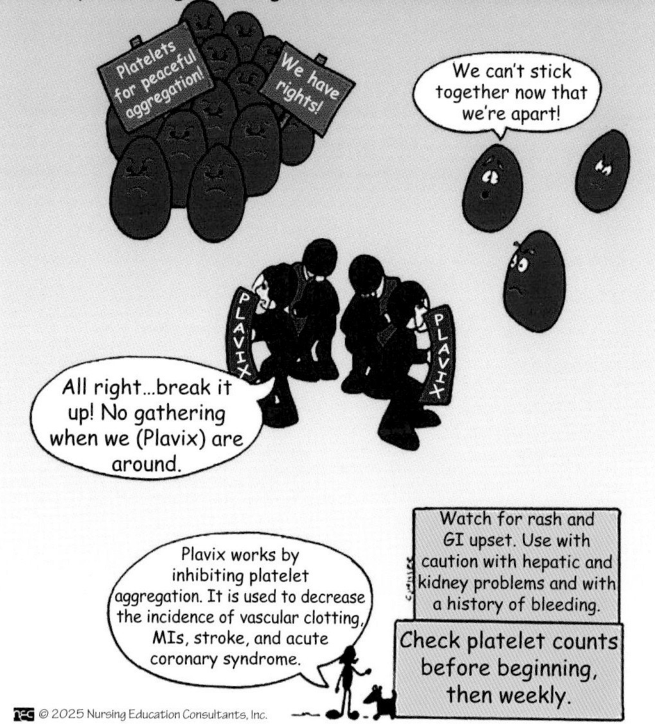

Platelets for peaceful aggregation!

We have rights!

We can't stick together now that we're apart!

PLAVIX

PLAVIX

All right...break it up! No gathering when we (Plavix) are around.

Plavix works by inhibiting platelet aggregation. It is used to decrease the incidence of vascular clotting, MIs, stroke, and acute coronary syndrome.

Watch for rash and GI upset. Use with caution with hepatic and kidney problems and with a history of bleeding.

Check platelet counts before beginning, then weekly.

What You Need to Know

Clopidogrel (Plavix)

CLASSIFICATION

Antiplatelet

ACTION ■ Black Box Warning ▲ High Alert

Suppresses platelet aggregation in arterial circulation; antiplatelet action occurs within 2 hours of administration.

USES

- Prevents occlusion of coronary stents
- Prevents/reduces thrombotic problems, such as MI, ischemic stroke, peripheral arterial disorders
- Secondary prevention of atherothrombotic events in patients with acute coronary syndromes, defined as unstable angina or MI

CONTRAINDICATIONS AND PRECAUTIONS

- Active bleeding, bleeding ulcers
- Hypersensitivity, breast-feeding, kidney and hepatic disease

SIDE EFFECTS

- Abdominal pain, dyspepsia, diarrhea (concern with GI bleeding)
- Bleeding—epistaxis, purpura, thrombotic thrombocytopenic purpura (TTP)
- Rash

NURSING IMPLICATIONS

1. May administer with food to diminish GI upset.
2. Teach patient to report any unusual bleeding or bruising (hematuria, tarry stools, epistaxis).
3. Teach patient that if surgery is scheduled, medication may be held 5 days before surgery.
4. Platelet counts may be monitored.
5. Teach patient to notify all HCPs regarding taking the medication.
6. Should not be taken with proton pump inhibitors (PPIs)—omeprazole (Prilosec); unless the patient has risk factors for GI bleeding (advanced age, use of nonsteroidal anti-inflammatory drugs, or anticoagulants), in which case pantoprazole (Protonix) is the preferred PPI. The benefits of combining a PPI with clopidogrel usually outweigh any risk from reduced antiplatelet effects.

Important nursing implications	Serious/life-threatening implications
Most frequent side effects	Patient teaching

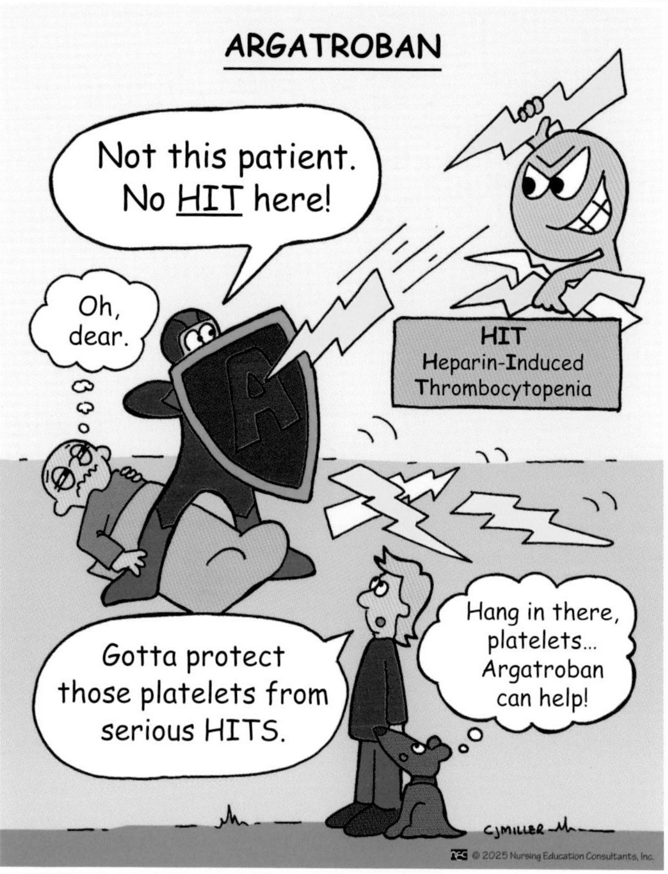
ARGATROBAN
Not this patient. No HIT here!
Oh, dear.
HIT Heparin-Induced Thrombocytopenia
Hang in there, platelets... Argatroban can help!
Gotta protect those platelets from serious HITS.
CJMILLER
© 2025 Nursing Education Consultants, Inc.

What You Need to Know

Argatroban

CLASSIFICATION

Anticoagulant

ACTION ▲ High Alert

Directly inhibits the action of thrombin in the clotting mechanism.

USES

- Prevents and treats HIT; prevents HIT during percutaneous coronary intervention (PCI)

CONTRAINDICATION

- Any evidence of overt bleeding

PRECAUTIONS

- Severe hypertension, hepatic impairment (dose adjusted)
- Recent major surgery
- Spinal anesthesia or lumbar puncture
- History of any bleeding disorders or intracranial bleeding

SIDE EFFECTS

- Allergic reactions: dyspnea, cough, rash—primarily in patients receiving other thrombolytic drugs or contrast media
- Hypotension, fever, diarrhea
- Bleeding episodes—hematemesis, hematuria, epistaxis, tarry stools, petechiae

NURSING IMPLICATIONS

1. Carefully monitor patient for any evidence of bleeding.
2. Monitor platelet count.
3. Administer only IV.
4. Dose and rate of administration are based on body weight.
5. Obtain baseline aPTT to monitor treatment. The aPTT returns to base level in 2 to 4 hours after medication is stopped. Dosage is adjusted to maintain the aPTT at 1.5 to 3 times the baseline value.

Important nursing implications | Serious/life-threatening implications
Most frequent side effects | Patient teaching

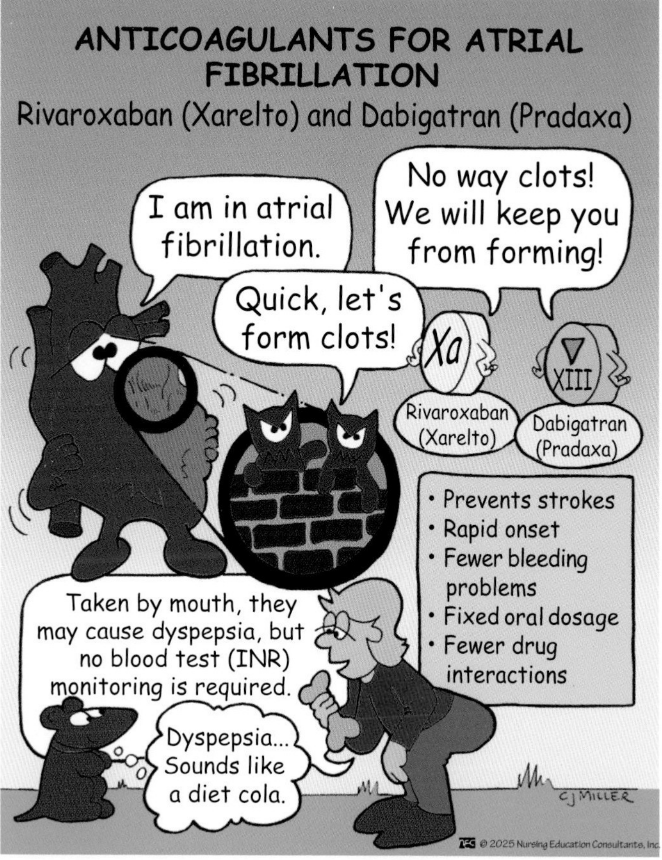
ANTICOAGULANTS FOR ATRIAL FIBRILLATION
Rivaroxaban (Xarelto) and Dabigatran (Pradaxa)
I am in atrial fibrillation.
No way clots! We will keep you from forming!
Quick, let's form clots!
Xa
XIII
Rivaroxaban (Xarelto)
Dabigatran (Pradaxa)
• Prevents strokes
• Rapid onset
• Fewer bleeding problems
• Fixed oral dosage
• Fewer drug interactions
Taken by mouth, they may cause dyspepsia, but no blood test (INR) monitoring is required.
Dyspepsia... Sounds like a diet cola.
CJ MILLER
© 2025 Nursing Education Consultants, Inc.

What You Need to Know

Anticoagulants for Atrial Fibrillation

DABIGATRAN, RIVAROXABAN, APIXABAN, EDOXABAN

Classification

Anticoagulant

- Dabigatran etexilate (Pradaxa): direct thrombin inhibitor
- Rivaroxaban (Xarelto): direct factor Xa inhibitor
- Apixaban (Eliquis): direct factor Xa inhibitor
- Edoxaban (Savaysa): direct factor Xa inhibitor

ACTIONS ■ Black Box Warning

Dabigatran

Directly inhibits thrombin formation, prevents conversion of fibrinogen to fibrin, prevents activation of factor XIII, and prevents the conversion of soluble fibrin into insoluble fibrin.

Rivaroxaban, Apixaban, Edoxaban

Inhibits production of thrombin by binding directly with factor Xa.

USES

- Prevent strokes and systemic embolism in patients with atrial fibrillation that is not related to a cardiac valve problem

PRECAUTIONS

- Pregnancy, active bleeding episodes, patients undergoing spinal puncture and/or epidural anesthesia
- Should not be combined with other anticoagulants; concurrent use with antiplatelet drugs and fibrinolytics should be done with caution (especially with rivaroxaban)
- Patients with severe kidney or hepatic disease (especially with rivaroxaban)

SIDE EFFECTS

- Bleeding, GI disturbances—dyspepsia, gastritis-like syndrome (with dabigatran)
- Spinal/epidural hematoma, permanent paralysis

NURSING IMPLICATIONS

1. Does not require monitoring by aPTT or INR levels.
2. Evaluate and monitor patient for bleeding risks.
3. Apixaban antidote: andexanet alfa (Andexxa); dabigatran antidote: idarucizumab (Praxbind).
4. Patient should be taught to take a missed dose as soon as possible, but not within 6 hours of next scheduled dose.
5. Dabigatran—should be used within 30 days after opening; it is sensitive to moisture and should not be stored in weekly pill organizers.
6. Take with food to decrease gastric side effects.

CALCIUM CHANNEL BLOCKERS & BETA BLOCKERS

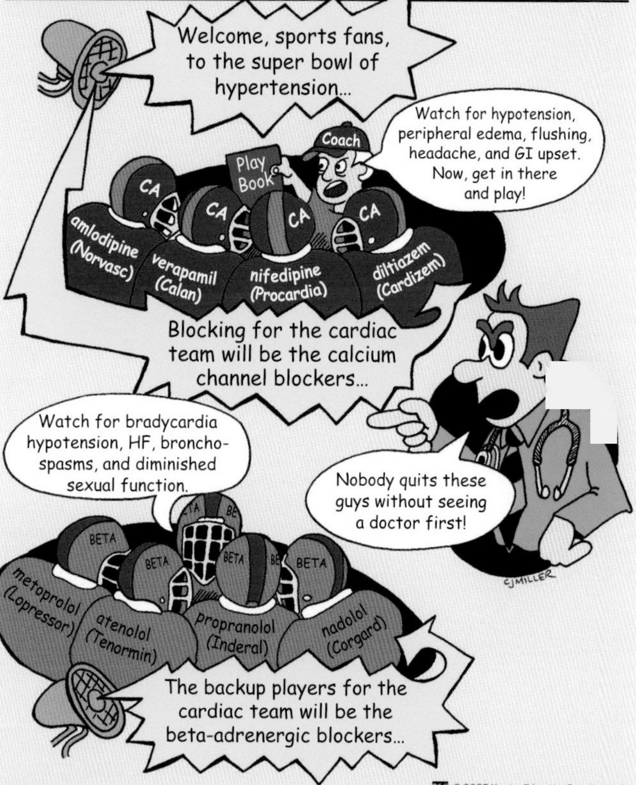

Welcome, sports fans, to the super bowl of hypertension...

Watch for hypotension, peripheral edema, flushing, headache, and GI upset. Now, get in there and play!

Coach

Play Book

CA

amlodipine (Norvasc)

verapamil (Calan)

nifedipine (Procardia)

diltiazem (Cardizem)

Blocking for the cardiac team will be the calcium channel blockers...

Watch for bradycardia hypotension, HF, broncho-spasms, and diminished sexual function.

Nobody quits these guys without seeing a doctor first!

BETA

metoprolol (Lopressor)

atenolol (Tenormin)

propranolol (Inderal)

nadolol (Corgard)

The backup players for the cardiac team will be the beta-adrenergic blockers...

CJMILLER

What You Need to Know

Calcium Channel Blockers and Beta-Blockers

ACTIONS

Antihypertensive drugs act on the vascular, cardiac, kidney, and sympathetic nervous systems. They act to lower blood pressure (BP), cardiac output (CO), and peripheral vascular resistance (PVR).

USES

- Control hypertension
- Angina pectoris, cardiac dysrhythmias
- Hypertensive emergency

CONTRAINDICATIONS

- Hypersensitivity
- Arterial stenosis
- Cerebrovascular insufficiency
- Severe bradycardia, atrioventricular (AV) heart block

PRECAUTIONS

- Uncontrolled heart failure, thyrotoxicosis
- Beta-blockers can mask symptoms of hypoglycemia in patients with diabetes
- Hepatic and kidney dysfunction

SIDE EFFECTS

- Hypotension, sedation
- Calcium channel blockers (CCBs)—bradycardia, peripheral edema, constipation, reflex tachycardia with nifedipine
- Beta-blockers—bradycardia, decreased AV conduction, reduced cardiac contractility, hypoglycemia, bronchoconstriction ■ Black Box Warning ▲ High Alert

NURSING IMPLICATIONS

1. Monitor vital signs.
2. Teach patients about orthostatic hypotension for initial dosing (e.g., get up slowly) and other lifestyle changes—weight reduction, sodium restriction, reduce alcohol consumption, smoking cessation, and daily exercise.
3. Monitor electrolyte, hepatic, and kidney serum blood studies.
4. Avoid abrupt withdrawal of drug; may cause rebound phenomenon of excessive rise in BP.
5. Verapamil and diltiazem—do not drink grapefruit juice when taking medication.

Important nursing implications | Serious/life-threatening implications

Most frequent side effects | Patient teaching

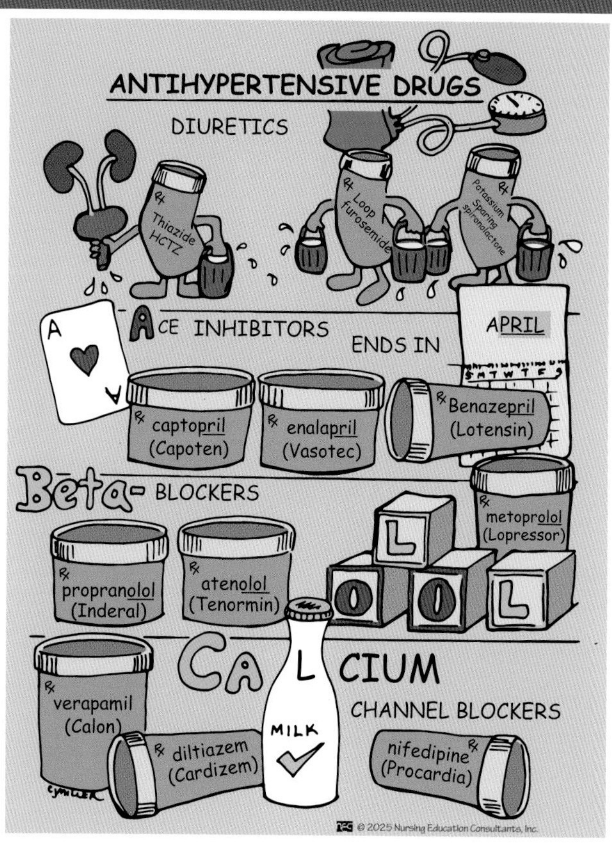
ANTIHYPERTENSIVE DRUGS
DIURETICS
Rx Thiazide HCTZ
Rx Loop furosemide
Rx Potassium Sparing spironolactone
ACE INHIBITORS
ENDS IN
APRIL
Rx captopril (Capoten)
Rx enalapril (Vasotec)
Rx Benazepril (Lotensin)
Beta- BLOCKERS
Rx propranolol (Inderal)
Rx atenolol (Tenormin)
Rx metoprolol (Lopressor)
L O L O L
CALCIUM
CHANNEL BLOCKERS
Rx verapamil (Calon)
Rx diltiazem (Cardizem)
MILK
Rx nifedipine (Procardia)
© 2025 Nursing Education Consultants, Inc.

What You Need to Know

Antihypertensive Drugs

CLASSIFICATION

BP is regulated by CO and PVR. Medications that influence either one of these systems lead to BP control. Antihypertensive drugs that influence these systems to lower BP are diuretics, angiotensin-converting enzyme (ACE) inhibitors, beta-adrenergic blockers, and calcium channel blockers (CCBs).

ACTIONS

- **A**—ACE inhibitors block the conversion of angiotensin I to angiotensin II, a vasoconstrictor. This block causes vasodilation and therefore decreases PVR, resulting in a decrease in BP. Aldosterone is also blocked, causing a decrease in sodium and water retention. ■ Black Box Warning
- **B**—Beta-adrenergic blockers block the $beta_1$-receptors in the heart, which results in decreased heart rate and decreased force of contraction. ■ Black Box Warning ▲ High Alert
- **C**—CCBs block calcium influx into beta-receptors, decrease the force of myocardial contraction, reduce heart rate, and decrease PVR.
- **D**—Diuretics, such as hydrochlorothiazide (HCTZ), are the first-line drugs for hypertension because they reduce blood volume (by diuresis) and decrease arterial resistance.

USES

- Control hypertension
- Either as separate drugs or frequently in combination with another drug

NURSING IMPLICATIONS

1. Initial drug selection starts with a thiazide diuretic (HCTZ), typically followed by a beta-adrenergic blocker or an ACE inhibitor or CCB.
2. Take medication as prescribed; do not stop abruptly.
3. Teach patients never to double up on doses if a dose is missed.
4. Change positions slowly; watch for postural hypertension.
5. Avoid over-the-counter medications.
6. Take caution in hot weather, hot showers, hot tub baths, or prolonged sitting or standing because these may aggravate low BP.
7. Teach patients about multidrug therapy; instruct them not to discontinue a previous antihypertensive medication when another medication is started.

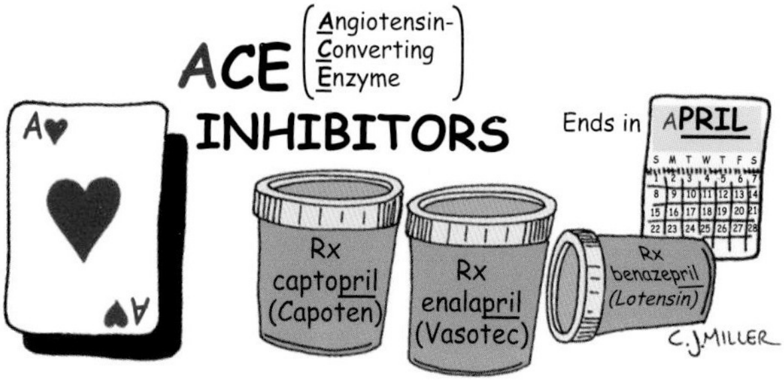

Actions: ↓ Peripheral vascular resistance **without:**

↑ Cardiac output
↑ Cardiac rate
↑ Cardiac contractility

Side Effects: Dizziness
Orthostatic hypotension
Fetal injury
Cough
Headache
Hyperkalemia

What You Need to Know

Angiotensin-Converting Enzyme (ACE) Inhibitors

ACTIONS ■ Black Box Warning

Blocks *production* of angiotensin II from the renin-angiotensin-aldosterone system, reduces peripheral resistance, and improves CO.

USES

- Hypertension, heart failure, myocardial infarction (MI)
- Diabetic and nondiabetic nephropathy

CONTRAINDICATIONS

- History of angioedema
- Pregnancy
- Bilateral renal artery stenosis

PRECAUTIONS

- Kidney failure, collagen vascular disease
- Hypovolemia, salt depletion

SIDE EFFECTS

- Postural hypotension (especially the first dose), headache, dizziness
- Nagging, dry, irritating, nonproductive cough
- Rash, angioedema
- Hyperkalemia
- Neutropenia (mainly with captopril)

NURSING IMPLICATIONS

1. Closely monitor BP, especially for 2 hours after the first dose, because severe first-dose hypotension often develops.
2. Teach patient to rise slowly from a lying to a sitting position to reduce postural hypotensive effects.
3. Before administering, assess the patient for history or presence of kidney impairment.
4. Administer on an empty stomach for best absorption.
5. Teach patient to notify health care provider (HCP) if cough develops.
6. Teach patient to avoid potassium supplements or potassium-containing salt substitutes.
7. Monitor kidney function and complete blood count and differential.

ATROPINE SIDE EFFECTS

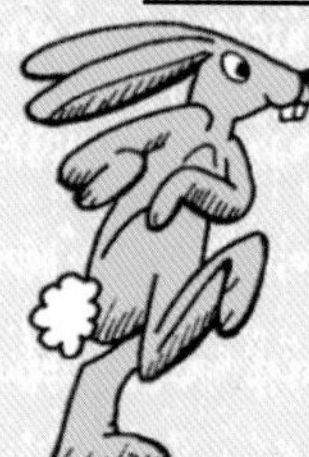

Hot as a Hare
(↑ temperature)

Mad as a Hatter
(confusion, delirium)

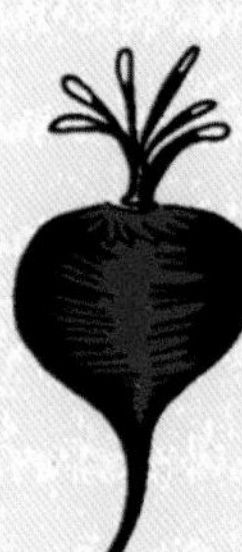

Red as a Beet
(flushed face)

Dry as a Bone
(decreased secretions, thirsty)

What You Need to Know

Atropine Side Effects

CLASSIFICATION

Anticholinergic, muscarinic antagonist

ACTION ▲ High Alert

Inhibits action of acetylcholine. Primary effects are on the heart, exocrine glands, smooth muscles, and eye.

USES

- Increases heart rate in symptomatic bradycardia, AV block
- Preoperative—decreases secretions
- Promotes mydriasis for retinal examination
- Decreases intestinal hypertonicity and hypermotility (diarrhea), biliary colic
- Muscarinic agonist poisoning (e.g., bethanechol, cholinesterase inhibitors)

PRECAUTIONS AND CONTRAINDICATIONS

- Gastrointestinal (GI) problems—obstruction, ulcers, colitis, gastroesophageal reflux disease
- Glaucoma, tachycardia, bladder obstruction (benign prostatic hyperplasia [BPH])
- Hyperthyroid, liver or kidney disease, asthma, hypertension
- On the Beers List—avoid use in the geriatric patient

ADVERSE EFFECTS

- Decreased sweating, which can lead to hyperthermia and flushing
- Central nervous system (CNS)—toxic doses may cause delirium and hallucinations
- Dry mouth (xerostomia), tachycardia
- Blurred vision, photophobia, urinary retention, urinary hesitancy, constipation

NURSING IMPLICATIONS

1. Evaluate hydration status; dry mouth relieved by sipping fluids and chewing sugar-free gum.
2. Evaluate frequently for urinary retention.
3. Do not administer if patient has tachycardia.
4. Teach patients to wear sunglasses outdoors.

Important nursing implications

Serious/life-threatening implications

Most frequent side effects

Patient teaching

POTASSIUM CHLORIDE (IV and PO)

Life Hangs in the Balance

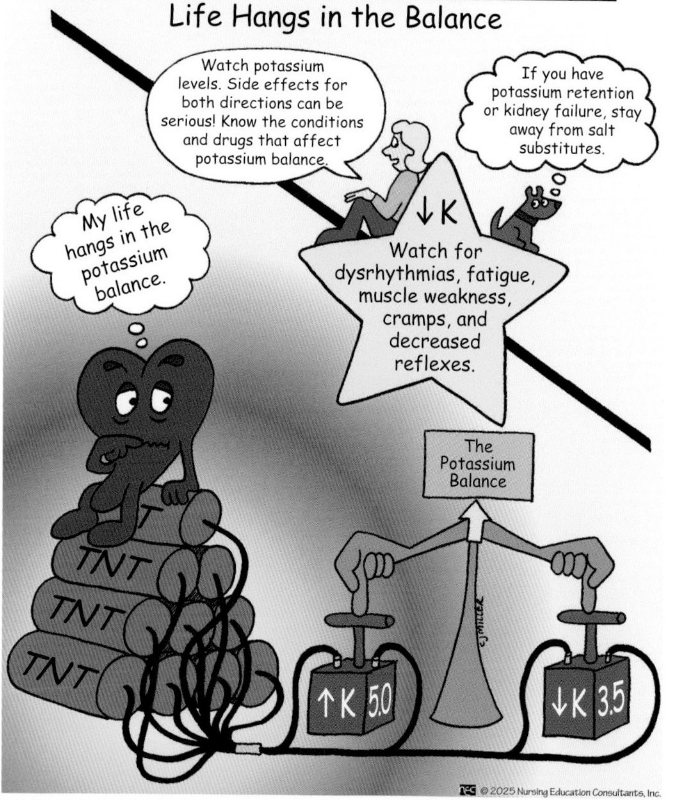

Watch potassium levels. Side effects for both directions can be serious! Know the conditions and drugs that affect potassium balance.

If you have potassium retention or kidney failure, stay away from salt substitutes.

My life hangs in the potassium balance.

↓K

Watch for dysrhythmias, fatigue, muscle weakness, cramps, and decreased reflexes.

The Potassium Balance

TNT

TNT

TNT

TNT

↑K 5.0

↓K 3.5

What You Need to Know

Potassium Chloride (Intravenous and Oral)

CLASSIFICATION

Electrolyte replacement

ACTIONS ▲ High Alert

Necessary for nerve impulse conduction; maintains electrical excitability of the heart and assists in regulating acid-base balance.

USES

- Prevents and/or corrects potassium deficiency

CONTRAINDICATIONS

- Hyperkalemia, use of potassium-sparing diuretics, hypoaldosteronism
- Kidney impairment
- Untreated Addison disease

PRECAUTIONS

- Acute acidosis resulting in potassium shifts
- ACE inhibitors

SIDE EFFECTS

- GI discomfort—nausea, vomiting, diarrhea
- Hyperkalemia—(primarily from intravenous [IV] infusion of potassium) ventricular fibrillation, cardiac dysrhythmias, cardiac arrest, confusion, anxiety, dyspnea, weakness, tingling

NURSING IMPLICATIONS

1. Give oral medication with a full glass of water with or after meals.
2. Sustained-release tablets (Klor-Con, Micro-K) are preferred because they are convenient and better tolerated.
3. Advise patient to take tablets whole; do not break, crush, split, or dissolve tablets.
4. Monitor serum potassium level.
5. Watch for signs of renal insufficiency—increased creatinine and increased blood urea nitrogen values; stop potassium and notify HCP if symptoms of kidney failure develop.
6. IV potassium *must always be diluted* before administering. **Never administer potassium via IV push.**
7. IV rate via a peripheral line is 10 mEq/hr and 20 to 40 mEq/hr via a central line.

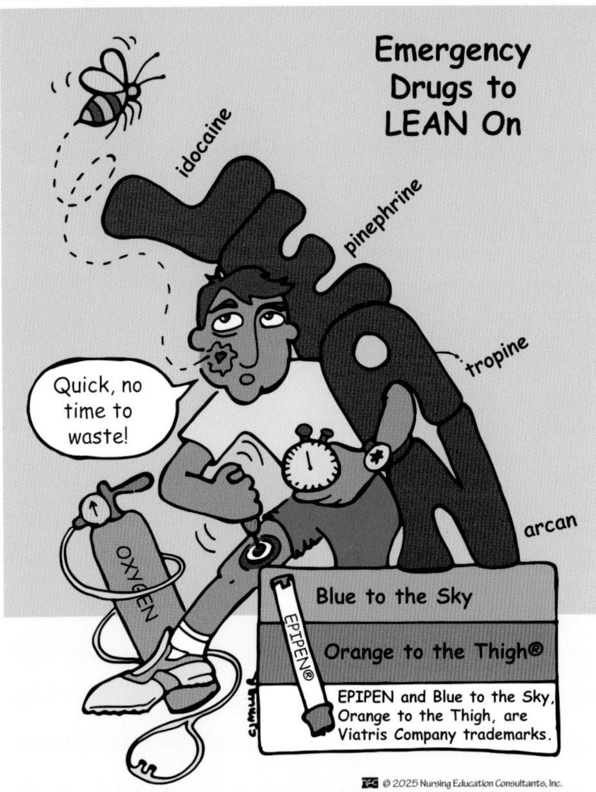
Emergency Drugs to LEAN On
idocaine
pinephrine
tropine
arcan
Quick, no time to waste!
OXYGEN
EPIPEN®
Blue to the Sky
Orange to the Thigh®
EPIPEN and Blue to the Sky, Orange to the Thigh, are Viatris Company trademarks.
© 2025 Nursing Education Consultants, Inc.

What You Need to Know

Emergency Drugs

LIDOCAINE

Antidysrhythmic, local anesthetic
Slows conduction, reduces automaticity, and increases repolarization of cardiac cycle. As an anesthetic, lidocaine causes temporary loss of feeling and sensation in the localized tissue.

Uses

IV preparation only for ventricular dysrhythmias (frequent premature ventricular beats, ventricular tachycardia)

EPINEPHRINE (ADRENALINE)

Adrenergic agonist, catecholamine ▲ **High Alert**
Causes vasoconstriction; increases heart rate and BP; is a bronchodilator; is the treatment of choice for anaphylactic reactions

Uses

For bronchodilation in patients with acute asthma; to treat hypersensitivity, anaphylactic reactions, cardiac arrest

ATROPINE

Anticholinergic, antidysrhythmic
Selectively blocks cholinergic receptors; increases heart rate in bradycardia; decreases secretions

Uses

To treat symptomatic bradycardia; to decrease respiratory secretions; to reverse effects of anticholinesterase medications

AMIODARONE (CORDARONE)

Antidysrhythmic ■ **Black Box Warning** ▲ **High Alert**
Decreases AV and sinus node function; suppresses dysrhythmias

Uses

Ventricular tachycardia and fibrillation

NALOXONE (NARCAN)

Opioid antagonist
Blocks narcotic effects; reverses opiate-induced sleep or sedation; increases respiratory rate and BP

Uses

Treatment of opioid overdose (morphine, meperidine, OxyContin); treats opioid-induced respiratory depression; may be used in neonates to counteract or treat effects from opioids given to mother during labor; used postoperatively to reverse respiratory and CNS depression

CA+LCIUM CHANNEL BLOCKERS

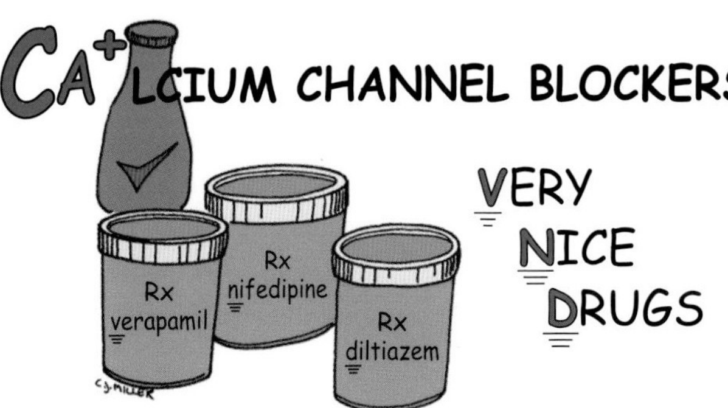

VERY
NICE
DRUGS

Actions: Block calcium access to cells causing:
- ↓ Contractility
- ↓ Conductivity of the heart
- ↓ Demand for oxygen

Side Effects:
- ↓ BP
- Bradycardia
- May precipitate AV block
- Headache
- Abdominal discomfort (constipation, nausea)
- Peripheral edema

What You Need to Know

Calcium Channel Blockers

ACTIONS

Block calcium access to the cells, causing decreased heart contractility and conductivity and leading to a decreased demand for oxygen; promote vasodilation.

USES

- Angina, hypertension, and dysrhythmias (verapamil and diltiazem)

CONTRAINDICATIONS

- *Nifedipine:* reflex tachycardia
- *Verapamil:* severe left ventricular dysfunction, decreased BP, cardiogenic shock, or heart block
- *Diltiazem:* sick sinus syndrome, heart block, decreased BP, acute MI, or pulmonary congestion

PRECAUTIONS

- Kidney or hepatic insufficiency may develop.
- Avoid giving verapamil or diltiazem with beta-blockers and digoxin.

SIDE EFFECTS

- Decreased BP, edema of the extremities, headache, reflex tachycardia (nifedipine)
- Constipation (verapamil), nausea, skin flushing (nifedipine, verapamil), dysrhythmias

NURSING IMPLICATIONS

1. Administer before meals; may be taken with food if needed; do not crush or allow patient to chew sustained-release medication preparations.
2. Monitor vital signs and watch for low BP.
3. Teach about postural hypotension and to notify HCP of signs of edema (swelling in ankles or feet).
4. Check liver and kidney function studies.
5. Weigh patient; report any peripheral edema or weight gain.
6. Teach patient to avoid grapefruit juice.
7. Teach patient that constipation can be minimized by increasing dietary fiber and fluid.
8. Teach patient to notify HCP of symptoms of slow heartbeat, shortness of breath, or weight gain.

ANGIOTENSIN II RECEPTOR BLOCKERS (ARBs)

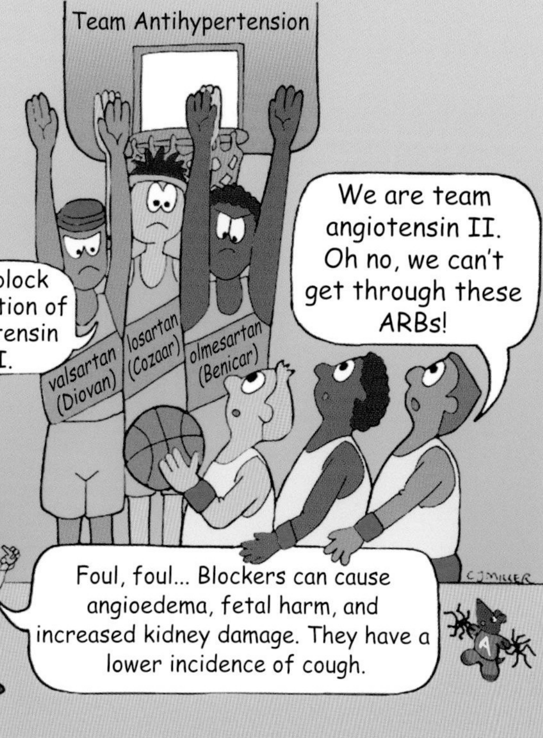

Team Antihypertension

We block the action of angiotensin II.

valsartan (Diovan)

losartan (Cozaar)

olmesartan (Benicar)

We are team angiotensin II. Oh no, we can't get through these ARBs!

Foul, foul... Blockers can cause angioedema, fetal harm, and increased kidney damage. They have a lower incidence of cough.

CJ MILLER

What You Need to Know

Angiotensin II Receptor Blockers (ARBs)

ACTIONS

Blocks the *action*, but not the production, of angiotensin II. Blocks the access of angiotensin II to its receptors in the heart, blood vessels, and adrenals, causing vasodilation.

USES

- Hypertension
- Heart failure (valsartan, candesartan), MI (valsartan)
- Diabetic nephropathy (irbesartan, losartan)
- Diabetic retinopathy for type 1 diabetes (losartan)
- Stroke prevention (losartan)
- Risk reduction in MI, stroke, and death from cardiovascular causes in patients aged 55 years and older if intolerant to ACE inhibitor (telmisartan)

CONTRAINDICATIONS

- Pregnancy and lactation
- Bilateral/unilateral renal artery stenosis; kidney failure
- History of angioedema
- Concurrent use with aliskiren (Tekturna) in patients with type 2 diabetes

SIDE EFFECTS

- Angioedema—can be severe and life-threatening
- Fetal injury during second and third trimesters
- Lower incidence of cough
- Kidney failure if renal artery stenosis is present

NURSING IMPLICATIONS

1. Monitor effect of medication on BP.
2. Assess for angioedema on initial administration—discontinue immediately if it occurs.
3. Monitor kidney function.
4. Monitor electrolyte levels, intake and output, and obtain daily weight—especially patients who are taking a combination drug containing an angiotensin receptor blocker plus a thiazide diuretic.
5. Review patient's medications—has an additive effect; dosages of the other antihypertensive drugs may require reduction.

NITROGLYCERIN

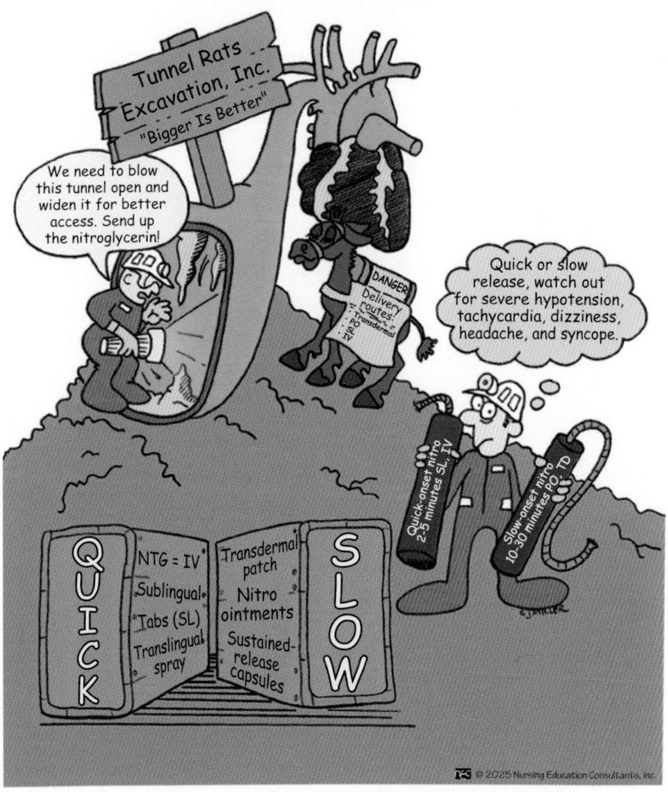

What You Need to Know

Nitroglycerin

ACTIONS

Is a vasodilator that relaxes vascular smooth muscle (arterial and venous) system with more prominent effects on veins, which decreases preload. The modest arteriolar relaxation reduces systemic vascular resistance, which decreases afterload. These actions decrease cardiac oxygen demand.

USES

- To relieve acute anginal pain and prevent further anginal pain

CONTRAINDICATIONS AND PRECAUTIONS

- Hypersensitive patients
- Erectile dysfunction medications (sildenafil [Viagra], tadalafil [Cialis], avanafil [Stendra], vardenafil [Levitra])—may lead to life-threatening hypotension
- Severe hepatic or kidney disease and use of other vasodilators
- Beta-blockers, verapamil, diltiazem

SIDE EFFECTS

- Orthostatic hypotension, headache, reflex tachycardia

NURSING IMPLICATIONS

1. Patients with angina should carry nitroglycerin with them at all times.
2. Teach proper storage for freshness (tingling, fizzle sensation under tongue). Discard unused medication after 24 months.
3. When angina occurs, teach patient to take a sublingual tablet (place under tongue); if pain is not relieved in 5 minutes, call 9-1-1. May take one tablet every 5 minutes for a total of three tablets while waiting for emergency care.
4. Avoid alcoholic beverages during nitroglycerin therapy.
5. Avoid swallowing or chewing sustained-release tablets to help drug reach GI system.
6. Rotate transdermal patches and remove after 12 to 14 hours to have a "patch-free" interval of 10 to 12 hours daily.
7. In hospitalized patients, check BP before administering.
8. Teach to direct the translingual spray against the oral mucosa; warn patient not to inhale the spray and to lie down before using.

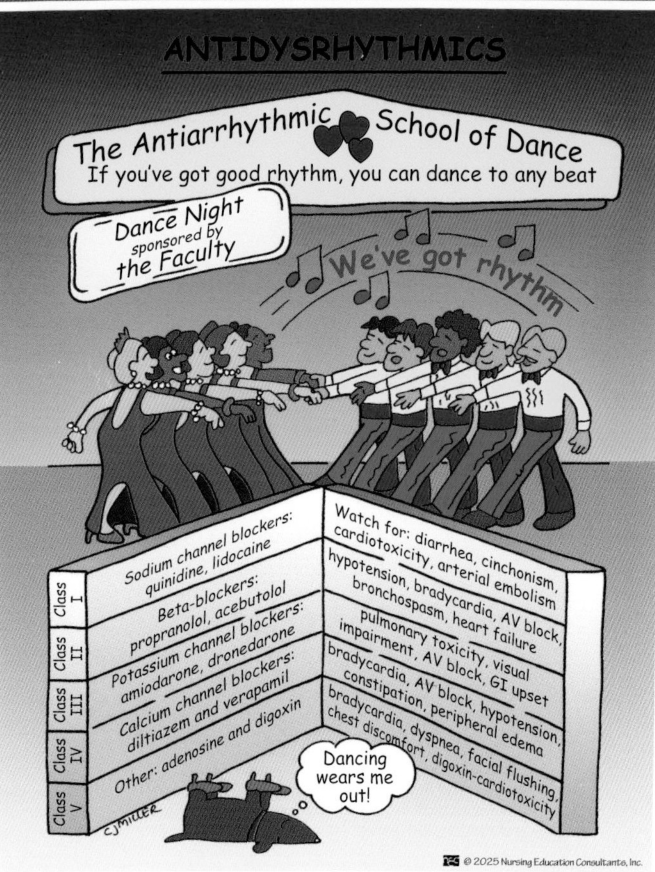
ANTIDYSRHYTHMICS
The Antiarrhythmic School of Dance
If you've got good rhythm, you can dance to any beat
Dance Night sponsored by the Faculty
We've got rhythm
Class I
Class II
Class III
Class IV
Class V
Sodium channel blockers: quinidine, lidocaine
Beta-blockers: propranolol, acebutolol
Potassium channel blockers: amiodarone, dronedarone
Calcium channel blockers: diltiazem and verapamil
Other: adenosine and digoxin
Watch for: diarrhea, cinchonism, cardiotoxicity, arterial embolism
hypotension, bradycardia, AV block, bronchospasm, heart failure
pulmonary toxicity, visual impairment, AV block, GI upset
bradycardia, AV block, hypotension, constipation, peripheral edema
bradycardia, dyspnea, facial flushing, chest discomfort, digoxin-cardiotoxicity
Dancing wears me out!
CJMILLER
© 2025 Nursing Education Consultants, Inc.

What You Need to Know

Antidysrhythmics

ACTIONS

- *Sodium channel blockers* block sodium, slowing the impulse in the atria, ventricles, and nodal and Purkinje systems (quinidine, lidocaine).
- *Beta-adrenergic blockers* reduce automaticity in the sinoatrial (SA) node, slow conduction velocity in the AV node, reduce contractility in the atria and ventricles (propranolol), and prolong the PR interval.
- *Potassium channel blockers* delay repolarization of fast potentials, prolong action potential duration and effective refractory period (amiodarone), and prolong the QT interval.
- *CCBs* block calcium channels and reduce the automaticity in the SA node, delay conduction through the AV node, delay reduction of myocardial contractility (diltiazem, verapamil), and prolong the PR interval.
- Adenosine and digoxin decrease conduction through the AV node and reduce automaticity of the SA node.

USES

- Tachydysrhythmia: supraventricular tachycardia (SVT), paroxysmal atrial tachycardia, atrial fibrillation

PRECAUTIONS

- Use with great caution in patients with AV block, bradycardia; medications can cause new dysrhythmias as well as exacerbate existing ones.

SIDE EFFECTS

- Quinidine: cinchonism effects—tinnitus, headaches, nausea, vomiting, dizziness
- Hypotension, fatigue, bradycardia
- Amiodarone—pulmonary toxicity, visual impairment, cardiotoxicity, photosensitivity, thyroid toxicity (hypo- or hyperthyroidism), liver toxicity

NURSING IMPLICATIONS

1. Monitor cardiac rhythm, particularly during initial dose for effectiveness; report apical pulse rate less than 60 beats per minute.
2. Report changes in dysrhythmias or occurrence of new one; assess for hypotension.
3. Instruct patient to take all prescribed doses and not to catch up on missed doses.
4. Instruct patient to report shortness of breath; pain; and irregular, fast, or slow heart rate.

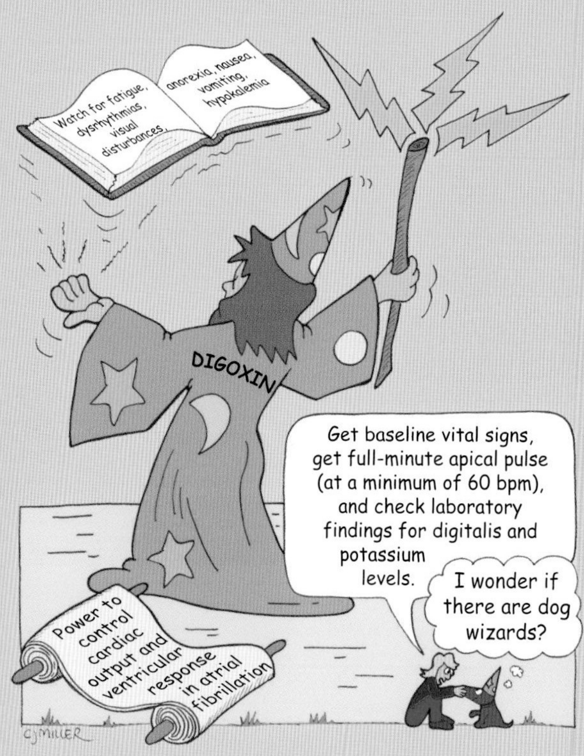
WIZARD OF DIGOXIN
Watch for fatigue, dysrhythmias, visual disturbances,
anorexia, nausea, vomiting, hypokalemia
DIGOXIN
Get baseline vital signs, get full-minute apical pulse (at a minimum of 60 bpm), and check laboratory findings for digitalis and potassium levels.
I wonder if there are dog wizards?
Power to control cardiac output and ventricular response in atrial fibrillation
CJMILLER
© 2025 Nursing Education Consultants, Inc.

What You Need to Know

Digoxin

ACTIONS ▲ High Alert

Affects the mechanical and electrical actions of the heart, which increases myocardial contractility (the force of ventricular contraction) and CO. Alters the electrical activity in the noncontractile tissue and ventricular muscle (e.g., automaticity, refractoriness, impulse conduction). Inhibits Na-K ATPase. Is classified as a cardiac glycoside.

USES

- Heart failure—to improve CO
- Atrial fibrillation and flutter
- Supraventricular dysrhythmias (SVT)

CONTRAINDICATIONS AND PRECAUTIONS

- Hypersensitivity, ventricular tachycardia, ventricular fibrillation, digoxin toxicity
- Renal insufficiency, hypokalemia, advanced heart failure, partial AV block, pregnancy
- When given with amiodarone, can increase digoxin level

SIDE EFFECTS

- Dizziness, headache, malaise, fatigue
- Nausea, vomiting, confusion, visual disturbances (blurred or yellow vision; halos around dark objects), anorexia—frequently foreshadow serious toxicity
- Hypokalemia (most common reason for digoxin-related dysrhythmias is diuretic-induced hypokalemia), dysrhythmias, bradycardia

NURSING IMPLICATIONS

1. Monitor digoxin serum levels; check for toxicity (2 ng/mL is considered toxic). Digoxin has a narrow therapeutic range.
2. Monitor pulse and teach patients to take their pulse. Report a pulse rate less than 60 or greater than 100 beats per minute for adults and rates less than 100 beats per minute for pediatric patients: hold the dose and notify a primary HCP.
3. Administer IV doses slowly over 5 minutes.
4. Teach patients to not double up with missed doses.
5. Teach patients to recognize early signs of hypokalemia (muscle weakness) and digoxin toxicity (nausea, vomiting, anorexia, diarrhea, blurred or yellow visual disturbances, halos around dark objects) and notify HCP.
6. Treatment of life-threatening digoxin toxicity/overdose is with IV DigiFab. Cholestyramine and activated charcoal bind digoxin and given orally to suppress absorption of digoxin in the GI tract.

LIDOCAINE TOXICITY

S — Slurred or difficult speech
- Paresthesias
- Numbness of lips/tongue

A — Altered cardiovascular system
- Drowsiness
- Dizziness
- Dysrhythmias
- Restlessness
- Hypotension
- Bradycardia, heart block

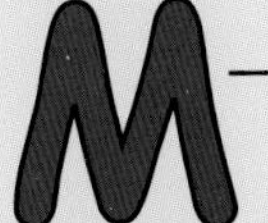

— Muscle twitching
- Tremors

S — Seizures
- Respiratory depression
- Respiratory and cardiac arrest

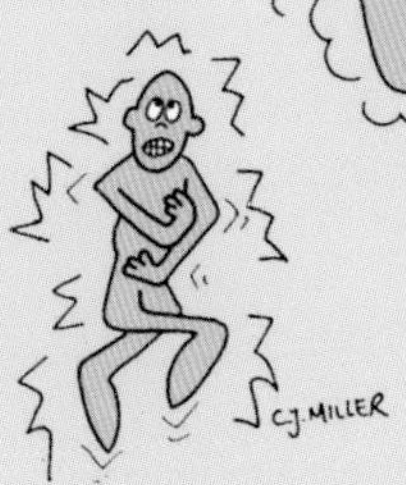

What You Need to Know

Lidocaine Toxicity

PATHOPHYSIOLOGY ▲ High Alert

Lidocaine is rapidly metabolized by the liver. If administered orally, the dose would be inactivated on the first pass through the liver. It is therefore given by IV infusion. Plasma drug levels are easily controlled. Its therapeutic range is 1.5 to 5.0 mcg/mL. In higher doses and at toxic levels, the central nervous and respiratory systems will be affected.

EFFECTS ON HEART AND ELECTROCARDIOGRAM

- Blocks sodium channels and slows conduction in the atria and ventricles
- Reduces automaticity in the ventricles and bundle of His-Purkinje system
- Accelerates repolarization
- No significant impact on electrocardiogram (ECG)

SIGNS AND SYMPTOMS OF TOXICITY

- High and prolonged doses—drowsiness, confusion, paresthesias
- Toxic doses—seizure, respiratory arrest

TREATMENT

- Equipment for resuscitation (crash cart) needs to be available.
- Seizures managed with diazepam or phenytoin.

NURSING IMPLICATIONS

1. Assess level of consciousness and orientation.
2. Administer at prescribed IV rate—administration that is too rapid can cause problems.
3. Protect for possible seizure activity; assess for paresthesia.
4. Check vital signs frequently.
5. Monitor ECG and report unusual activity or changes in rhythm.
6. Assess respiratory system, ventilation, and gas exchange (oxygen saturation).
7. Lidocaine preparations that contain epinephrine must never be administered IV; doing so can cause severe hypertension and life-threatening dysrhythmias. Lidocaine used for local anesthesia often contains epinephrine.

DRUGS FOR BRADYCARDIA AND DECREASED BLOOD PRESSURE

= IDEA

I SOPROTERENOL
D OPAMINE
E PINEPHRINE
A TROPINE

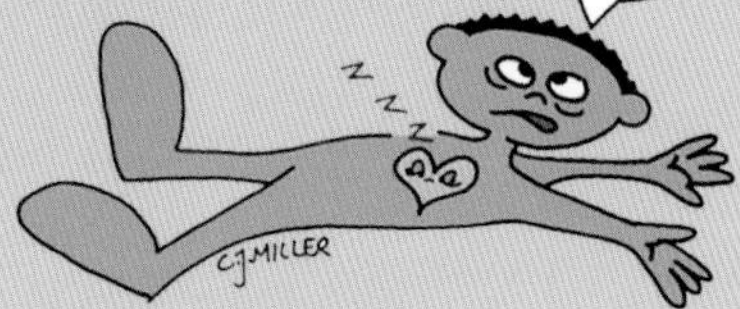

What You Need to Know

Drugs for Bradycardia and Decreased BP

ISOPROTERENOL (ISUPREL)

Classification
Sympathomimetic, catecholamine

ACTIONS ▲ High Alert
Increases heart rate and CO, causes bronchodilation

ADVERSE EFFECTS
Tachycardia and angina; can cause hyperglycemia in patients with diabetes

DOPAMINE

Classification
Sympathomimetic, catecholamine

ACTIONS ■ Black Box Warning ▲ High Alert
Low doses cause renal blood vessel vasodilation. Moderate doses increase cardiac contractility, stroke volume, and CO. Higher doses increase PVR, BP, and renal vasoconstriction.

ADVERSE EFFECTS
Tachycardia, dysrhythmias, anginal pain, vasoconstriction leading to tissue necrosis with extravasation (treatment for extravasation is phentolamine)

EPINEPHRINE (ADRENALINE)

Classification
Adrenergic agonist, catecholamine

ACTIONS ▲ High Alert
Causes vasoconstriction and increases heart rate; bronchodilator; treatment of choice for anaphylactic reactions.

ADVERSE EFFECTS
Hypertension, hypertensive crisis, dysrhythmias, anginal pain, restlessness, necrosis following extravasation, hyperglycemia in patients with diabetes

ATROPINE

Classification
Anticholinergic, antidysrhythmic

ACTIONS
Acts on smooth muscle of the heart and increases cardiac rate

ADVERSE EFFECTS
Tachycardia, palpitations, dry mouth (xerostomia), drowsiness, blurred vision, photophobia, urinary hesitancy/retention

ALPHA-ADRENERGIC ANTAGONISTS (ALPHA-BLOCKERS) SIDE EFFECTS

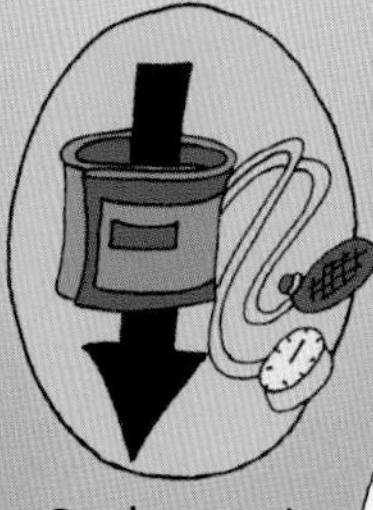

Orthostatic Hypotension

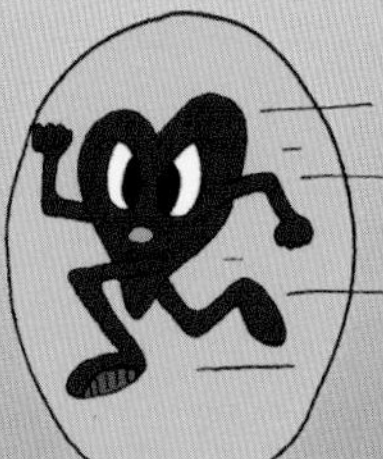

Reflex Tachycardia

Examples:

alfuzosin
doxazosin
prazosin
terazosin

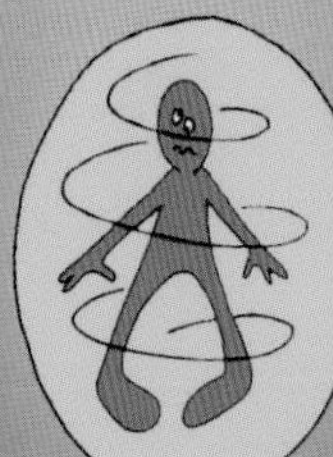

Dizziness

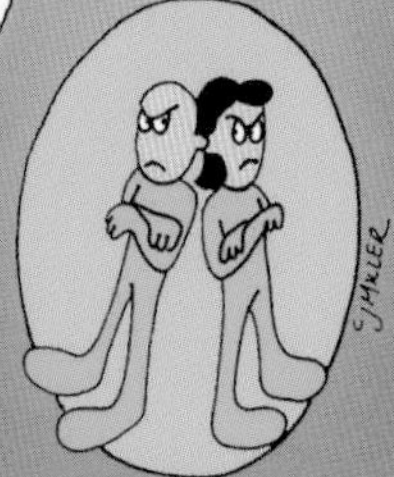

Sexual Dysfunction (inhibition of ejaculation)

What You Need to Know

Alpha-Adrenergic Antagonists (Alpha-Blockers) Side Effects

EXAMPLES

Alfuzosin, doxazosin, prazosin, tamsulosin, terazosin
(*Note: The suffix of **osin** and **zosin** for this group.*)

ACTIONS

Stimulate central alpha-receptors, which decreases sympathetic outflow from the CNS, causing a decrease in PVR and a slight decrease in CO. Relaxes smooth muscle in bladder neck, prostate capsule, and prostatic urethra; improves urine outflow in patients with benign prostatic hyperplasia (BPH).

USES

- Mild-to-moderate hypertension
- Reversal of toxicity from $alpha_1$ agonists—phentolamine is given
- BPH

PRECAUTIONS AND CONTRAINDICATIONS

- Hypersensitivity to drug and sulfites
- Patients with liver disease, blood dyscrasias, and pheochromocytoma

SIDE EFFECTS

- Orthostatic hypotension
- Reflex tachycardia, dizziness, drowsiness, sedation
- Inhibition of ejaculation, nasal congestion, dry mouth

NURSING IMPLICATIONS

1. Watch for orthostatic hypotension, which is intensified with prolonged standing, hot baths or showers, hot weather, alcohol use, and strenuous exercise.
2. Teach patient that they should consume no more than four cups of caffeinated coffee, tea, or cola per day.
3. Patient should take medicine at bedtime to avoid drowsiness during the day.
4. Discontinue slowly to avoid rebound hypertension.
5. Teach patient about the need for lifelong therapy if taking for BPH.
6. Teach patient about first-dose effect of severe orthostatic hypotension and to avoid hazardous activities and driving for 12 to 24 hours after initial dose. To decrease risk, instruct patient to take the first dose at bedtime.

BETA-ADRENERGIC ANTAGONISTS (BETA-BLOCKERS) SIDE EFFECTS

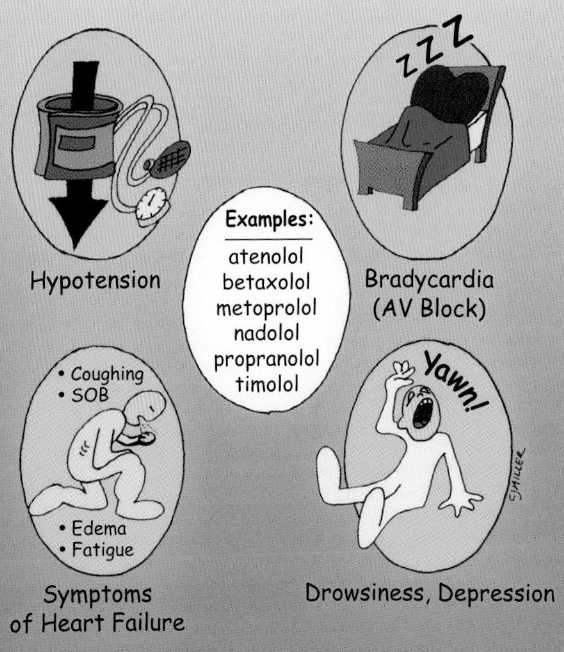

What You Need to Know

Beta-Adrenergic Antagonists (Beta-Blockers) Side Effects

EXAMPLES

Atenolol, betaxolol, propranolol, metoprolol, nadolol, timolol
(*Note: The suffix* ***olol*** *for this group.*)

ACTIONS ■ Black Box Warning ▲ High Alert

Block sympathetic nervous system catecholamines, resulting in reduced renin and aldosterone release and fluid balance. Vasodilation of arterioles leads to a decrease in pulmonary vascular resistance and BP. Blockade leads to reduced heart rate, reduced force of contraction, and reduced velocity of impulse conduction through the AV node.

USES

- Hypertension, antianginal agents in long-term treatment of angina
- Dysrhythmias—to suppress sinus and atrial tachydysrhythmias
- MI, hyperthyroidism, migraine prophylaxis, pheochromocytoma, glaucoma
- Carvedilol, bisoprolol, and metoprolol are considered effective for heart failure

CONTRAINDICATIONS

- AV block (if greater than first degree), bradydysrhythmias, severe allergies

PRECAUTIONS

- Can cause bronchoconstriction; use with caution in patients with diabetes (masks signs of hypoglycemia), kidney or hepatic dysfunction
- History of depression
- Avoid during pregnancy; caution with breast-feeding

SIDE EFFECTS

- Postural hypotension, bradycardia, drowsiness, sleep disturbance (nightmares), depression, heart failure
- Bronchospasm, bronchoconstriction, malaise, lethargy

NURSING IMPLICATIONS

1. Assess vital signs; monitor closely if given with a CCB.
2. Report any weakness, dizziness, bradycardia, or fainting.
3. Report any edema or difficulty breathing.
4. Monitor patients with diabetes; increased risk of hypoglycemia—tachycardia (a symptom of hypoglycemia) is often masked because of the $beta_1$ blockade.

HMG-CoA REDUCTASE INHIBITORS (Antihyperlipidemics)

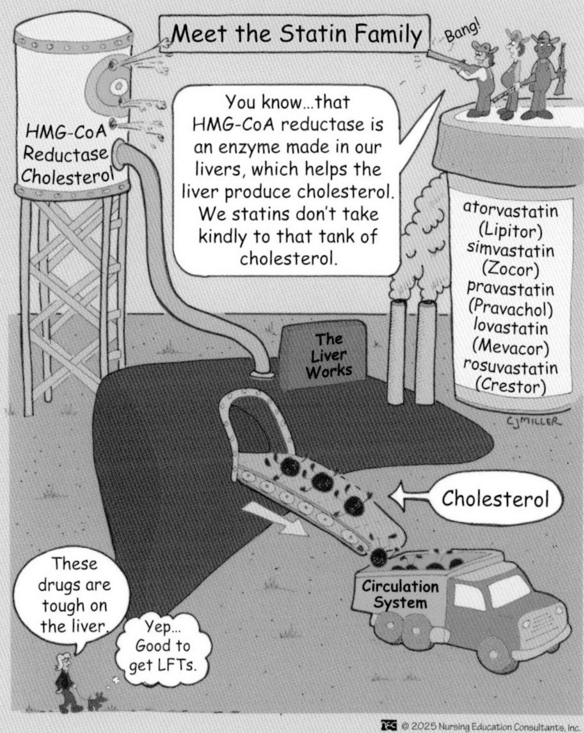

What You Need to Know

HMG-CoA Reductase Inhibitors (Statins)

EXAMPLES

Atorvastatin, fluvastatin, simvastatin, pravastatin, lovastatin, rosuvastatin

ACTION

Lower cholesterol levels by inhibiting the formation of HMG-CoA reductase, which is an enzyme that is required for the liver to synthesize cholesterol. Effective in decreasing low-density lipoprotein and increasing high-density lipoprotein levels and may lower triglycerides in some patients.

USES

- Hypercholesterolemia
- Primary and secondary prevention of cardiovascular events
- Patients with type 2 diabetes and coronary heart disease

CONTRAINDICATIONS

- Viral or alcoholic hepatitis; pregnancy

PRECAUTIONS

- Liver disease, depending on severity
- Excessive alcohol use

SIDE EFFECTS

- Headache, rash, or GI disturbances (dyspepsia, cramps, flatulence, constipation, abdominal pain)
- Myopathy—myositis, rhabdomyolysis (severe form; rarely occurs)
- Hepatotoxicity—liver injury with increases in levels of serum transaminases

NURSING IMPLICATIONS

1. Instruct patient to report unexplained muscle pain or tenderness.
2. Monitor liver function studies.
3. Inform women of childbearing age about the potential for fetal harm should they become pregnant.
4. Administer medication in the evening without regard to meals, except for lovastatin, which is taken with the evening meal (extended-release tablet taken at bedtime).
5. Instruct patient about dietary changes to reduce weight and cholesterol.

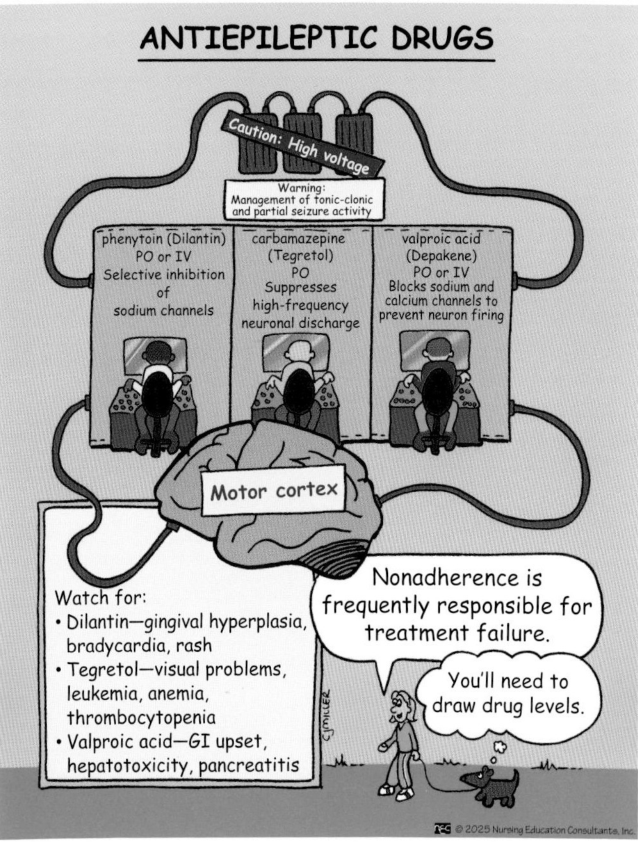
ANTIEPILEPTIC DRUGS
Caution: High voltage
Warning:
Management of tonic-clonic and partial seizure activity
phenytoin (Dilantin) PO or IV Selective inhibition of sodium channels
carbamazepine (Tegretol) PO Suppresses high-frequency neuronal discharge
valproic acid (Depakene) PO or IV Blocks sodium and calcium channels to prevent neuron firing
Motor cortex
Watch for:
• Dilantin—gingival hyperplasia, bradycardia, rash
• Tegretol—visual problems, leukemia, anemia, thrombocytopenia
• Valproic acid—GI upset, hepatotoxicity, pancreatitis
Nonadherence is frequently responsible for treatment failure.
You'll need to draw drug levels.
CJMILLER
© 2025 Nursing Education Consultants, Inc.

What You Need to Know

Antiepileptic Drugs

ACTIONS ■ Black Box Warning

Suppresses discharge of neurons within a seizure focus area and decreases spread of seizure activity to other areas of the brain

USES

- Medications are specific to type of seizure (generalized or partial) and to specific categories of seizures.
- Can be used for status epilepticus.

CONTRAINDICATIONS

- Hypersensitivity
- Pregnancy (teratogenic effects)

PRECAUTIONS

- Hepatic, hematologic, respiratory disorders
- Sinus bradycardia, sinoatrial block, second- and third-degree block (Dilantin)

SIDE EFFECTS

- Valproic acid (Depakote): constipation, nausea, vomiting, hepatotoxicity, fatal pancreatitis
- Carbamazepine (Tegretol): blood dyscrasias, visual disturbances, ataxia, vertigo
- Phenytoin (Dilantin): nystagmus, cognitive impairment, hypotension, gingival hyperplasia, measles-like rash, ataxia, extravasation at intravenous (IV) site

NURSING IMPLICATIONS

1. Usually given orally. Do not mix IV Dilantin with other medications. Give IV Dilantin slowly (do not exceed 50 mg/min) and monitor cardiac rhythm during IV administration.
2. Perform periodic blood studies for therapeutic levels.
3. Check hepatic and kidney functions.
4. Teach patient to purchase a Medic-Alert bracelet or carry a medical ID card.
5. Teach patient to never abruptly discontinue medication.
6. With Dilantin, watch for gingival hyperplasia; encourage routine prophylactic dental care and instruct patient to take with meals; suggest taking 0.5 mg of folic acid daily.
7. Do not give Tegretol with grapefruit juice.
8. Teach patient to report rash (Dilantin), signs of infection (Tegretol), signs of pancreatitis or liver injury (valproic acid).

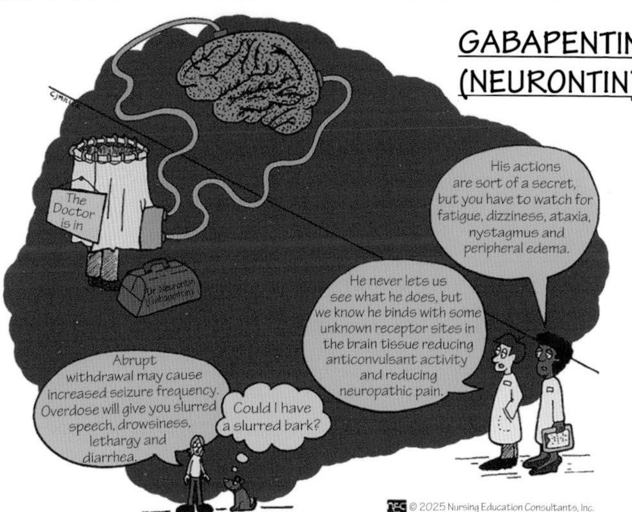
GABAPENTIN (NEURONTIN)
The Doctor is in
His actions are sort of a secret, but you have to watch for fatigue, dizziness, ataxia, nystagmus and peripheral edema.
He never lets us see what he does, but we know he binds with some unknown receptor sites in the brain tissue reducing anticonvulsant activity and reducing neuropathic pain.
Abrupt withdrawal may cause increased seizure frequency. Overdose will give you slurred speech, drowsiness, lethargy and diarrhea.
Could I have a slurred bark?
© 2025 Nursing Education Consultants, Inc.

What You Need to Know

Gabapentin (Neurontin)

ACTIONS

Reduces seizure activity and neuropathic pain; exact mechanism unknown

USES

- Approved for epilepsy as adjunctive therapy of focal seizures (with or without bilateral convulsion)
- Postherpetic neuralgia
- Off-label uses: neuropathic pain, diabetic neuropathy, prophylaxis of migraine, treatment of fibromyalgia, postmenopausal hot flashes

CONTRAINDICATIONS

- Hypersensitivity

PRECAUTIONS

- Two forms of gabapentin are *not currently indicated* for management of epilepsy.
  - Gabapentin ER (Gralise) is approved for management of postherpetic neuralgia.
  - Gabapentin enacarbil (Horizant) is approved for treatment of moderate-to-severe restless legs syndrome.
- These two forms of gabapentin *are not interchangeable* with each other or with Neurontin.

SIDE EFFECTS

- Somnolence, dizziness, ataxia, fatigue, nystagmus, peripheral edema.
- Overdosage may result in slurred speech, drowsiness, diarrhea, lethargy.
- Drug reaction with eosinophilia and systemic symptoms or multiorgan hypersensitivity can occur and is characterized by fever; rash; swollen, painful, or tender lymph glands; bleeding; jaundice.

NURSING IMPLICATIONS

1. Administer with or without food.
2. Administering the first dose at bedtime is preferred because it may cause excessive sleepiness.
3. Teach patient to never abruptly discontinue medication, as abrupt withdrawal may increase seizure frequency.
4. Teach patient who take antacids that contain aluminum or magnesium to wait at least 2 hours before taking gabapentin.
5. Teach patient to avoid driving and other hazardous activities until they are familiar with drug's side effects.

PROMETHAZINE (PHENERGAN)

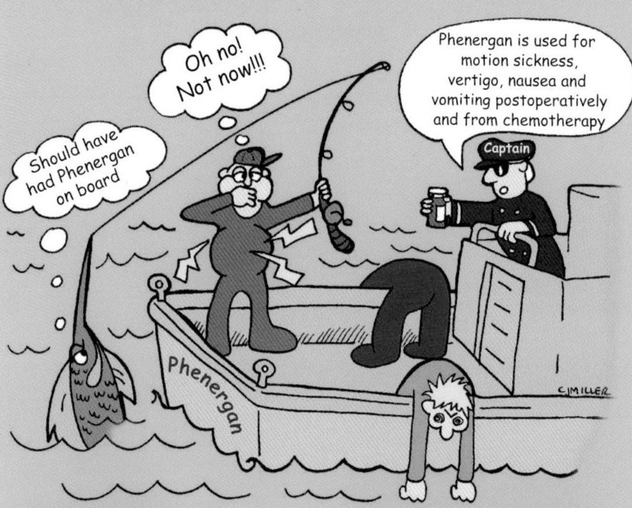

Delivery

PO
PR
IM
IV

Watch for:

- Drowsiness
- Restlessness
- Hypotension
- Confusion
- Urinary retention

What You Need to Know

Promethazine (Phenergan)

CLASSIFICATION

Antiemetic (dopamine antagonist-phenothiazine); antihistamine

ACTION ■ Black Box Warning ▲ High Alert

Blocks dopamine receptors in the chemoreceptor trigger zone (CTZ)

USES

- Nausea and vomiting, motion sickness
- Preoperative and postoperative sedation

CONTRAINDICATIONS AND PRECAUTIONS

- Children less than 2 years old—fatal respiratory depression
- Extreme caution in children more than 2 years old—seizures
- Glaucoma, gastrointestinal (GI), or genitourinary obstruction
- Pregnancy, seizures, asthma, severe central nervous system (CNS) depression; avoid use in the older adult

SIDE EFFECTS

- Sedation, drowsiness, disorientation
- Hypotension, syncope in the older adult
- Severe respiratory depression and risk of death, especially in children
- Dry mouth, urinary retention
- Epigastric distress, flushing, visual and hearing disturbances
- Extra pyramidal symptoms (EPS)—dystonia, akathiasia
- Neuroleptic malignant syndrome

NURSING IMPLICATIONS

1. Evaluate patient's respiratory status during use of this drug.
2. Teach patient to avoid tasks that require mental alertness; do not drink alcohol or take with CNS depressants.
3. Direct patient to report tremors or abnormal body movements.
4. Long-term therapy: teach patient to have complete blood count drawn.
5. If administered IV and extravasation occurs, severe tissue injury and necrosis can lead to gangrene or amputation of extremity, so deep intramuscular (IM) route is preferred. Teach patient to immediately report local burning or pain during IV therapy.
6. Evaluate older adult's ability to urinate.
7. Teach patient measures to reduce dry mouth.

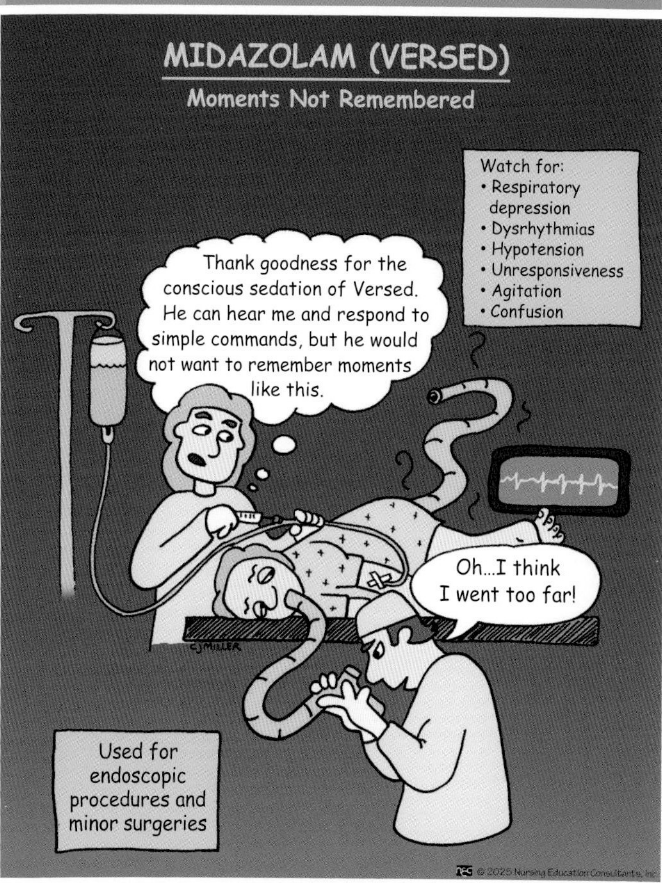
MIDAZOLAM (VERSED)
Moments Not Remembered
Watch for:
• Respiratory depression
• Dysrhythmias
• Hypotension
• Unresponsiveness
• Agitation
• Confusion
Thank goodness for the conscious sedation of Versed. He can hear me and respond to simple commands, but he would not want to remember moments like this.
Oh...I think I went too far!
Used for endoscopic procedures and minor surgeries
CJMILLER
© 2025 Nursing Education Consultants, Inc.

What You Need to Know

Midazolam (Versed)

CLASSIFICATION

Benzodiazepine

Other benzodiazepines administered for induction of anesthesia—diazepam, lorazepam

ACTION ■ Black Box Warning ▲ High Alert

Produces unconsciousness and amnesia

USES

- Induction of anesthesia and conscious sedation
- Management of acute seizures

CONTRAINDICATIONS

- Shock, coma, hypotension, acute alcohol intoxication, acute narrow-angle glaucoma

PRECAUTIONS

- Can cause dangerous cardiorespiratory effects, including respiratory depression and cardiac arrest
- Acute illness, severe electrolyte imbalance
- Increased sedation effects with ingestion of grapefruit juice
- Older adult patients with chronic obstructive pulmonary disease (COPD)

SIDE EFFECTS

- Decreased respiratory rate, tenderness at IM/IV injection site, hypotension
- Toxicity: slurred speech, impaired motor coordination, ataxia, coma, death

NURSING IMPLICATIONS

1. Administer slowly over 2 or more minutes. Wait another 2 or more minutes for full effects to develop before giving additional doses to avoid cardiorespiratory problems.
2. Unconsciousness develops quickly (within 60–80 seconds). Conscious sedation persists for approximately 1 hour.
3. Perform constant cardiac and respiratory monitoring during administration with resuscitative equipment nearby.
4. The patient may not remember any postoperative instructions. After outpatient procedures, the patient must be accompanied home by a responsible adult.
5. The patient should not operate a car or engage in activities requiring alertness for 24 hours after receiving medication.
6. Antidote for toxicity and overdose: flumazenil.

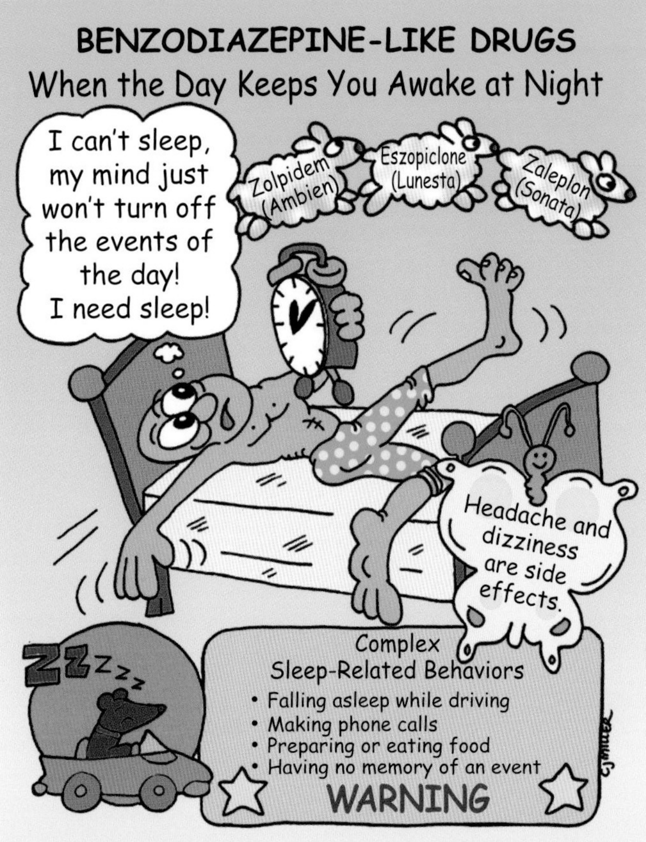
BENZODIAZEPINE-LIKE DRUGS
When the Day Keeps You Awake at Night
I can't sleep, my mind just won't turn off the events of the day! I need sleep!
Zolpidem (Ambien)
Eszopiclone (Lunesta)
Zaleplon (Sonata)
Headache and dizziness are side effects.
Complex Sleep-Related Behaviors
• Falling asleep while driving
• Making phone calls
• Preparing or eating food
• Having no memory of an event
WARNING
ZZZzzz
© 2025 Nursing Education Consultants, Inc.

What You Need to Know

Benzodiazepine-Like Drugs

ACTION

Act as agonist at the benzodiazepine receptor site on the gamma-aminobutyric acid receptor

USES

- Insomnia
  - Zolpidem (Ambien) and zaleplon (Sonata)—short-term treatment for insomnia
  - Eszopiclone (Lunesta)—no limitation on length of usage

CONTRAINDICATIONS AND PRECAUTIONS

- Pregnancy, lactation
- Hepatic impairment, depression, history of drug usage

SIDE EFFECTS

- Drowsiness, dizziness, confusion
- Bitter aftertaste (eszopiclone)
- Sleep-related complex behaviors—sleep driving, making phone calls, preparing food while asleep, having no memory of the activity
- Rebound insomnia may occur first evening after discontinuing drug

NURSING IMPLICATIONS

1. Is a Schedule IV substance—low potential for tolerance, dependence, or abuse.
2. Can intensify effects of other hypnotics and CNS depressants.
3. Teach patient to not break or chew the extended-release capsules.
4. Teach patient to not use medication in combination with alcohol.
5. Encourage patient to take the medication immediately before going to bed—do not participate in activities that require mental alertness.
6. Teach patient measures to enhance sleep—decreased consumption of caffeine-containing beverages (e.g., coffee, tea, colas), warm milk, bathing, quiet environment, reading, comfort measures.
7. Carefully assess effects on older adult patients.

ONDANSETRON (ZOFRAN)

(Serotonin Receptor Antagonist)

granisetron (Sancuso); dolasetron (Anzemet); palonosetron (Aloxi)

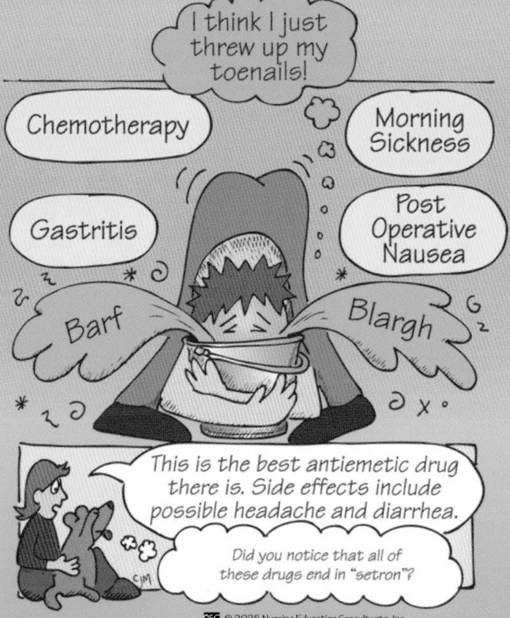

I think I just threw up my toenails!

Chemotherapy

Morning Sickness

Gastritis

Post Operative Nausea

Barf

Blargh

This is the best antiemetic drug there is. Side effects include possible headache and diarrhea.

Did you notice that all of these drugs end in "setron"?

What You Need to Know

Ondansetron (Zofran)

CLASSIFICATION

Antiemetic (serotonin receptor antagonist)

Other serotonin receptor antagonists are granisetron (Sancuso), dolasetron (Anzemet), palonosetron (Aloxi). *Note: All generic names end in "***setron.***"*

ACTIONS

Prevents nausea and vomiting by blocking type 3 serotonin receptors (5-HT receptors) located in the chemoreceptor trigger zone and on afferent vagal neurons in the upper GI tract. Does not cause extrapyramidal effects (e.g., akathisia, acute dystonia) as seen with phenothiazide antiemetics.

USES

- Chemotherapy-induced nausea and vomiting
- Anesthesia, postoperative nausea
- Radiation therapy
- Morning sickness of pregnancy
- Gastritis

CONTRAINDICATIONS AND PRECAUTIONS

- Children and older adult patients
- Patients with long QT syndrome
- Electrolyte abnormalities, heart failure
- Bradydysrhythmias

SIDE EFFECTS

- Headache, dizziness, drowsiness
- Diarrhea, constipation, abdominal pain
- Prolongs the QT interval (Zofran only) and poses a risk of torsades de pointes (life-threatening dysrhythmia)

NURSING IMPLICATIONS

1. Assess for effectiveness of medication—absence of nausea and vomiting during chemotherapy, anesthesia, gastritis, morning sickness of pregnancy.
2. Monitor for side effects—anticipate patient requiring an analgesic (e.g., acetaminophen) for headache.
3. Teach patient to report diarrhea, constipation, rash, changes in respiration, or discomfort at the injection site.
4. Administer IV piggyback preparations slowly over 15 minutes.

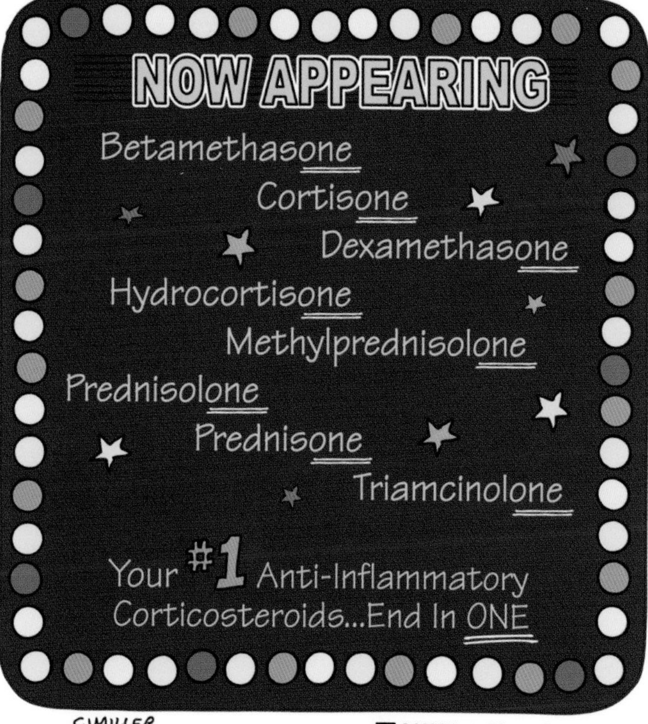
NOW APPEARING
Betamethasone
Cortisone
Dexamethasone
Hydrocortisone
Methylprednisolone
Prednisolone
Prednisone
Triamcinolone
Your #1 Anti-Inflammatory
Corticosteroids...End In ONE
CJMILLER
NEC © 2025 Nursing Education Consultants, Inc.

What You Need to Know

Corticosteroids

ACTION

Acts by suppressing inflammatory and immune responses. *Examples*: short acting (cortisone, hydrocortisone), intermediate acting (methylprednisolone, prednisolone, prednisone, triamcinolone), long acting (betamethasone, dexamethasone).

USES

- Suppress rejection of organ transplants and treatment of a variety of inflammatory, allergic, and neoplastic disorders, including rheumatoid arthritis, systemic lupus erythematosus, osteoarthritis, bursitis/tendinitis, inflammatory bowel disease, asthma
- Prevention of respiratory distress syndrome in preterm infants

CONTRAINDICATIONS

- Systemic fungal infections and patients receiving live virus vaccines

SIDE EFFECTS

- Adrenal insufficiency, osteoporosis, increased risk of infection
- Muscle wasting, thinning of the skin, fluid retention, and electrolyte imbalance (hypokalemia)
- Hyperglycemia, psychologic disturbances, peptic ulcer disease
- Long-term, high-dose therapy can cause fat redistribution, resulting in the central obesity (potbelly), moon face, and buffalo hump that characterize Cushing syndrome
- Cataracts and glaucoma with long-term therapy

NURSING IMPLICATIONS

1. Dose should be tapered very gradually when medication is discontinued.
2. Glucocorticoids may be prescribed every other day before 0900 to help minimize adrenal insufficiency and to mimic the normal release of the glucocorticoids by the adrenal glands each morning (alternate-day therapy).
3. Teach patient to carry identification (e.g., Medic-Alert bracelet).
4. Dosage is increased when stress occurs (e.g., surgery, trauma, infection).
5. Educate patient about signs and symptoms of *hypokalemia* (irregular pulses, muscle weakness/cramping, constipation) and *fluid retention* (weight gain, dependent edema) and instruct patient to notify health care provider (HCP) if these symptoms develop.
6. Teach patient to report to the HCP early signs of infection (e.g., fever, sore throat), if vision becomes blurred or cloudy, or if stools become black and tarry.
7. Teach women who are receiving high-dose therapy not to breast-feed.
8. Immunizations should not be administered while taking steroids.

Important nursing implications | Serious/life-threatening implications

Most frequent side effects | Patient teaching

CLOBETASOL

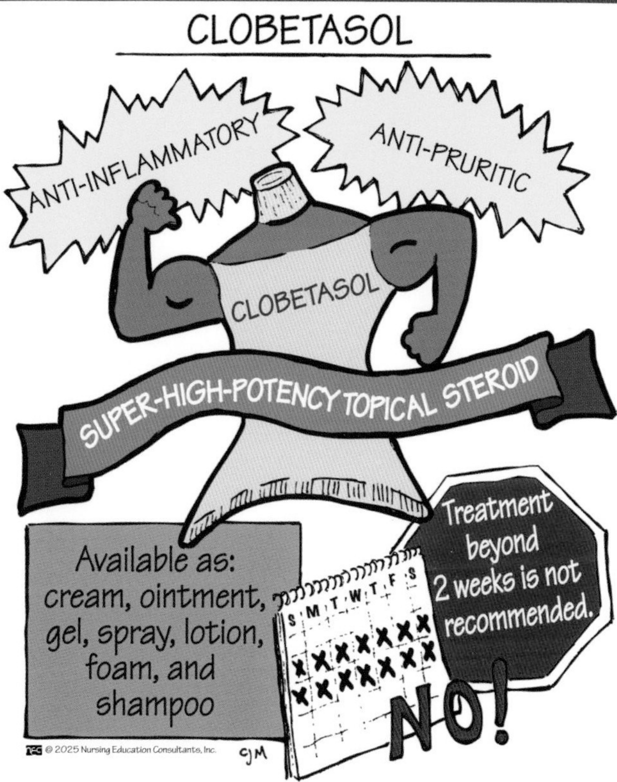

ANTI-INFLAMMATORY
ANTI-PRURITIC
CLOBETASOL
SUPER-HIGH-POTENCY TOPICAL STEROID
Available as: cream, ointment, gel, spray, lotion, foam, and shampoo
S M T W T F S
Treatment beyond 2 weeks is not recommended.
NO!
© 2025 Nursing Education Consultants, Inc.
CJM

What You Need to Know

Clobetasol

ACTION

Clobetasol is a super-high-potency topical glucocorticoid that is used to relieve inflammation and itching.

USES

- Dermatitis, psoriasis, eczema, pemphigus, insect bites

CONTRAINDICATIONS AND PRECAUTIONS

- Contraindicated for viral, fungal, or tubercular skin lesions
- Chronic topical corticosteroid therapy may interfere with growth and development in children
- May cause hypercorticism or suppression of hypothalamic-pituitary-adrenal (HPA) axis, especially in younger children or patients receiving high doses for prolonged periods
- Use with caution during pregnancy and breast-feeding

SIDE EFFECTS

- With prolonged use, atrophy of the dermis and epidermis, resulting in thinning of the skin, striae (stretch marks), purpura, telangiectasis, acne, excessive growth of hair, especially on the face
- Systemic toxicity: growth delay in children and adrenal suppression in all age groups

NURSING IMPLICATIONS

1. Topical glucocorticoids can be absorbed into the systemic circulation.
    - Absorption is higher where the skin is especially permeable (axilla, face, eyelids, neck, perineum, genitalia).
    - Lower rate of absorption from regions where penetrability is poor (palms, soles).
    - Absorption rate through intact skin is lower than through inflamed skin.
2. Apply topical medication after cleansing the area, dry well before applying a thin film of the medication.
3. Teach patient to avoid using occlusive dressings (bandages, plastic wraps) unless the HCP tells them to. This includes tight-fitting diapers, plastic pants, and disposable undergarments for urinary or bowel incontinence.

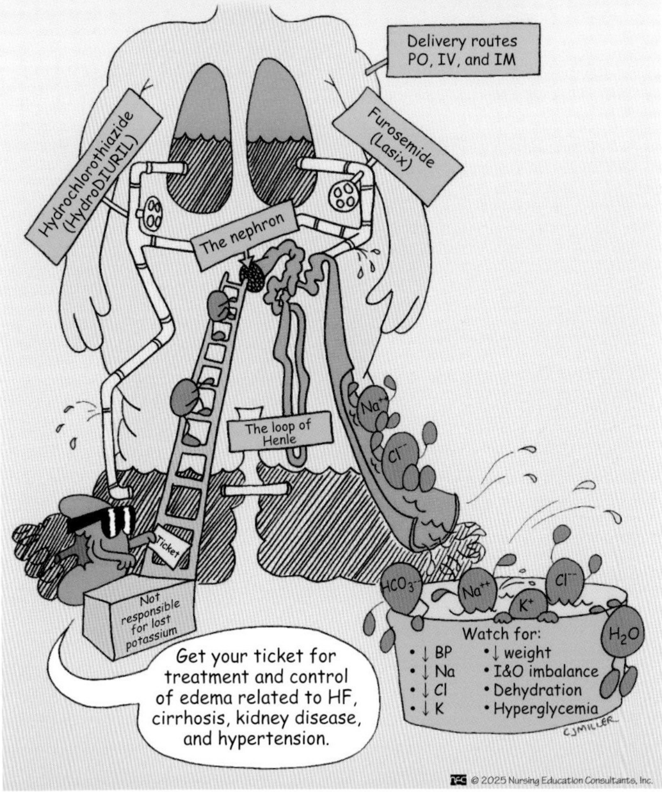
DIURETIC WATER SLIDE
Delivery routes PO, IV, and IM
Hydrochlorothiazide (HydroDIURIL)
Furosemide (Lasix)
The nephron
The loop of Henle
Na^{++}
Cl^{--}
Ticket
Not responsible for lost potassium
Get your ticket for treatment and control of edema related to HF, cirrhosis, kidney disease, and hypertension.
HCO_3^{--}
Na^{++}
K^+
Cl^{--}
H_2O
Watch for:
• ↓ BP
• ↓ Na
• ↓ Cl
• ↓ K
• ↓ weight
• I&O imbalance
• Dehydration
• Hyperglycemia
CJMILLER
© 2025 Nursing Education Consultants, Inc.

What You Need to Know

Diuretics

ACTIONS

Loop diuretics (furosemide) inhibit sodium (Na) and chloride (Cl) reabsorption through direct action primarily in the ascending loop of Henle but also in the proximal and distal tubules. *Thiazide diuretics* (hydrochlorothiazide [HCTZ]) act primarily on the distal convoluted tubule, inhibiting Na and Cl reabsorption.

USES

- To treat edema that involves fluid volume excess resulting from several disorders of the heart, liver, or kidney
- Hypertension

CONTRAINDICATIONS AND PRECAUTIONS

- Not recommended during pregnancy, breast-feeding
- Severe adrenocortical impairment
- Fluid and electrolyte depletion, gout
- Use with caution in patients taking digitalis, lithium, nonsteroidal anti-inflammatory drugs (NSAIDs), and other antihypertensive medications
- Caution and careful monitoring when administering a loop diuretic with another medication that is ototoxic, i.e., aminoglycosides

SIDE EFFECTS

- Dehydration, hyponatremia, hypochloremia, hypokalemia
- Unusual tiredness, weakness, dizziness
- Irregular heartbeat, weak pulse, orthostatic hypotension
- Tinnitus, hyperglycemia, hyperuricemia, hearing loss (loop diuretics)

NURSING IMPLICATIONS

1. Monitor for adequate intake and output and potassium loss.
2. Monitor patient's weight and vital signs.
3. Monitor for signs and symptoms of hearing loss with loop diuretics, which may last from 1 to 24 hours and irreversible hearing loss with ethacrynic acid.
4. Encourage patient to eat foods rich in potassium (sweet potatoes, dried fruits, spinach, nuts).
5. Teach patient to take medication early in the day to decrease nocturia.
6. Teach patient to report any hearing loss or signs of gout.

Important nursing implications | Serious/life-threatening implications
Most frequent side effects | Patient teaching

FUROSEMIDE (LASIX)

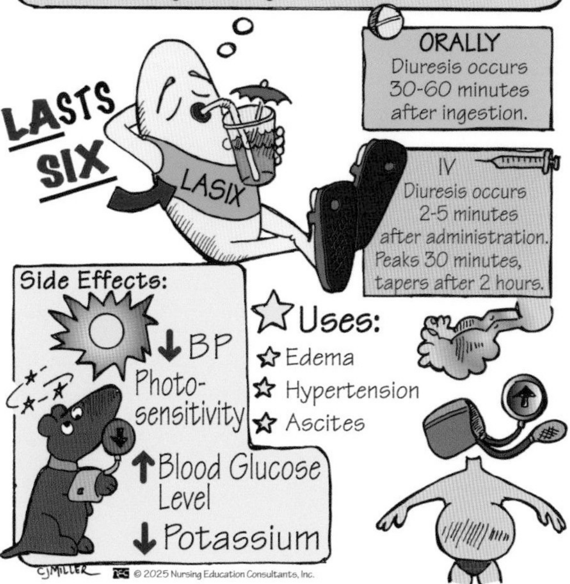

What You Need to Know

Furosemide (Lasix)

ACTIONS ■ Black Box Warning ▲ High Alert

Furosemide inhibits sodium (Na) and chloride (Cl) reabsorption through direct action primarily in the ascending loop of Henle but also in the proximal and distal tubules. Also known as a "high-ceiling" diuretic because it is more effective than other diuretics.

USES

- Pulmonary edema associated with heart failure (HF)
- Edema of hepatic, cardiac, or kidney origin that has been unresponsive to less efficacious diuretics
- Hypertension that cannot be controlled with other diuretics

CONTRAINDICATIONS AND PRECAUTIONS

- Not recommended during pregnancy, breast-feeding
- Severe adrenocortical impairment
- Fluid and electrolyte depletion, gout
- Use with caution in patients taking digitalis, ototoxic drugs, potassium-sparing diuretics, lithium, NSAIDs, and other antihypertensive medications

SIDE EFFECTS

- Severe dehydration (dry mouth, oliguria, increased thirst), thrombosis, embolism
- Hyponatremia, hypochloremia, hypokalemia
- Orthostatic hypotension (dizziness, lightheadedness, fainting).
- Hyperglycemia, hyperuricemia, transient hearing loss
- Reduces high-density lipoprotein cholesterol and raises low-density lipoprotein (LDL) cholesterol and triglycerides
- Photosensitivity
- Increase urinary excretion of calcium leading to hypocalcemia

NURSING IMPLICATIONS

1. Monitor for adequate intake and output and potassium loss.
2. Monitor patient's weight and vital signs.
3. Monitor for signs and symptoms of hearing loss.
4. Teach patient to take medication early in the day to decrease nocturia.
5. Teach patient to report any hearing loss or signs of gout.

HYDROCHLOROTHIAZIDE

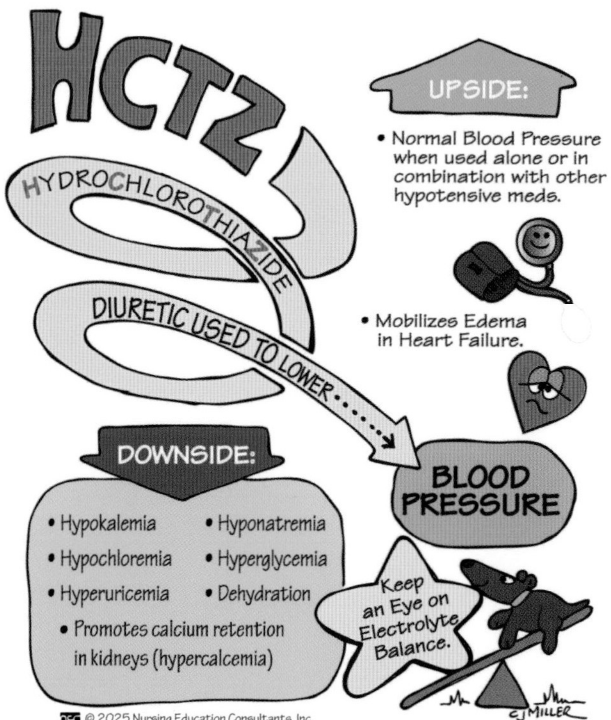

What You Need to Know

Hydrochlorothiazide

ACTIONS ▲ High Alert

HCTZ promotes urine production by blocking the reabsorption of sodium (Na) and chloride (Cl) in the early segment of the distal convoluted tubule. Therefore the patient must have adequate kidney function for the diuretic to be effective.

USES

- Essential hypertension
- Edema of hepatic, cardiac, or kidney origin
- Diabetes insipidus—reduce urine production by 30% to 50%; not clear on mechanism of this paradoxical effect
- Protection against postmenopausal osteoporosis by promoting tubular reabsorption of calcium

CONTRAINDICATIONS AND PRECAUTIONS

- Not recommended during pregnancy, breast-feeding
- History of hypersensitivity to sulfonamides
- Severe kidney impairment; glomerular filtration rate (GFR) <15 to 20 mL/min
- Severe adrenocortical impairment
- Fluid and electrolyte depletion, gout
- Use with caution in patients taking digitalis, ototoxic drugs, potassium-sparing diuretics, lithium, NSAIDs, and other antihypertensive medications

SIDE EFFECTS

- Hyponatremia, hypochloremia, hypokalemia, dehydration
- Orthostatic hypotension (dizziness, lightheadedness, fainting)
- Hyperglycemia, hyperuricemia, hypercalcemia
- Increases LDL cholesterol, total cholesterol, triglycerides
- Magnesium deficiency (hypomagnesemia)

NURSING IMPLICATIONS

1. Monitor for adequate intake and output and potassium loss.
2. Monitor patient's weight and vital signs.
3. Monitor for signs and symptoms of hearing loss.
4. Teach patient to take medication early in the day to decrease nocturia.
5. Teach patient to take medication with or after meals if gastrointestinal (GI) upset occurs.
6. Teach patient to report any signs of gout.

SPIRONOLACTONE
(Aldactone)

Water-In/Water-Out
Research Lab

Save the potassium—
get rid of the water! Blocks
action ofaldosterone in the kidney.
Gets rid of the sodium and water,
but saves the potassium.

Watch for:
- Hyperkalemia
- Headache/dizziness
- GI disturbances
- Fatigue
- Cramps

Spironolactone

Triamterene

Remember, too little
or too much potassium will
cause weakness in muscles,
including the heart.

What You Need to Know

Spironolactone (Aldactone)

CLASSIFICATION

Potassium-sparing diuretic

ACTIONS ■ Black Box Warning

Blocks the action of aldosterone in the distal nephron, which leads to retention of potassium and increased excretion of sodium. Effects of spironolactone are delayed, taking up to 48 hours to develop, so action is not immediate.

USES

- Treats hypertension and edema
- Reduces edema in patients with severe HF
- Primary hyperaldosteronism, premenstrual syndrome, polycystic ovary syndrome, acne in young women

CONTRAINDICATIONS

- Hypersensitivity or kidney failure
- Anuria
- Hyperkalemia

PRECAUTIONS

- Kidney and hepatic dysfunction

SIDE EFFECTS

- Hyperkalemia, dehydration
- Weakness, GI disturbances (bleeding), leg cramps
- Endocrine effects: hirsutism, menstrual irregularities, gynecomastia, impotence, deepening of voice

NURSING IMPLICATIONS

1. Monitor intake and output and watch for cardiac dysrhythmias.
2. Monitor levels of electrolytes (e.g., potassium, sodium); do not administer with potassium supplements or salt substitutes containing potassium chloride.
3. Teach patient to report leg cramps, weakness, fatigue, or nausea.
4. Teach patient to restrict intake of potassium-rich foods (e.g., nuts, dried fruits, spinach, citrus fruits, potatoes, bananas).
5. Teach patient to take medication with or after meals if GI upset occurs.
6. Have patient notify health care provider if menstrual irregularities, gynecomastia, or impotence occurs.
7. Because the medication may cause fetal harm, the nurse should wear a protective gown and two sets of gloves when cutting or crushing tablets.

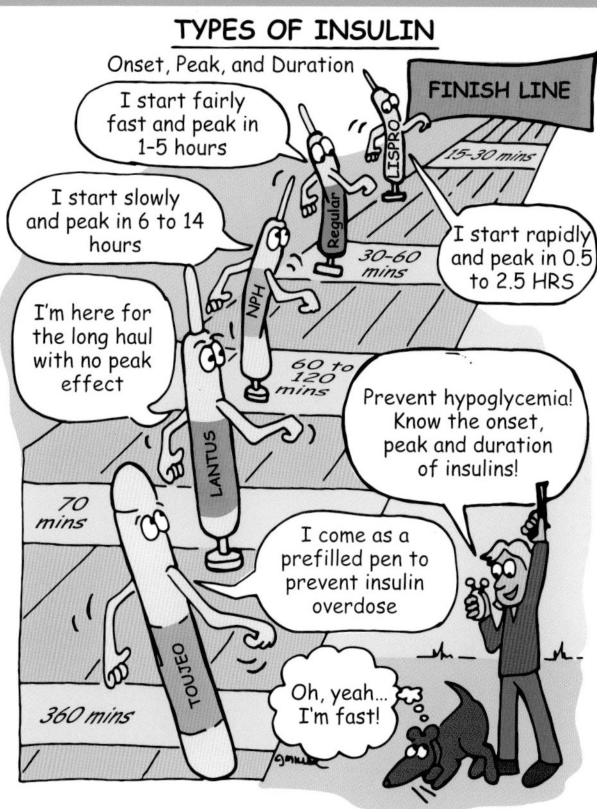
TYPES OF INSULIN
Onset, Peak, and Duration
FINISH LINE
I start fairly fast and peak in 1-5 hours
LISPRO
Regular
15-30 mins
I start slowly and peak in 6 to 14 hours
I start rapidly and peak in 0.5 to 2.5 HRS
30-60 mins
NPH
I'm here for the long haul with no peak effect
60 to 120 mins
Prevent hypoglycemia! Know the onset, peak and duration of insulins!
LANTUS
70 mins
I come as a prefilled pen to prevent insulin overdose
TOUJEO
360 mins
Oh, yeah... I'm fast!
© 2025 Nursing Education Consultants, Inc.

What You Need to Know

Types of Insulin

ACTIONS ■ Black Box Warning ▲ High Alert

	Onset (min)	Peak (h)	Duration (h)
Short Duration: Rapid Acting			
Insulin lispro (Humalog)	15–30	0.5–2.5	3–6
Insulin aspart (NovoLog)	10–20	1–3	3–5
Insulin glulisine (Apidra)	10–15	1–1.5	3–5
Short Duration: Short Acting			
Regular insulin (Humulin R, Novolin R)	30–60	1–5	6–10
Intermediate Duration			
NPH insulin (Humulin N, Novolin N)	60–120	6–14	16–24
Long Duration			
Insulin glargine (U-100) (Lantus)	70	None	18–24
Insulin detemir (Levemir)	60–120	None	12–24
Ultra-Long Duration			
Insulin glargine (U-300) (Toujeo)	360	None	>24
Insulin degludec (Tresiba)	30–90	None	>24

From Burchum, J. R., & Rosenthal, L. D. (2022). *Lehne's pharmacology for nursing care* (11th ed.). Elsevier.

NURSING IMPLICATIONS

1. U-100 insulin is the most common concentration.
2. Always use a U-100 insulin syringe with U-100 insulin.
3. NPH is the only cloudy insulin; roll the vial gently between palms to mix.
4. Draw up the clear (regular, lispro, aspart, and glulisine—short-acting or rapid-acting) insulin before the cloudy (NPH—intermediate duration) insulin to prevent contaminating a shorter-acting insulin with a longer-acting insulin.
5. Inject subcutaneously (abdomen, upper arm, thigh); aspiration is not necessary.
6. Avoid massaging the site after injection.
7. Rotate sites within anatomic area (about 1 inch apart); the abdomen is preferred for more rapid, even absorption. Inject 2 inches away from the umbilicus and avoid injecting near surgical sites, drains, wounds, or open skin areas.
8. Only NPH (Humulin N) can be mixed with rapid-acting or short-acting insulins.
9. While rapid- and short-acting insulin may be administered intravenously (IV), only regular insulin (Humulin R) is usually given IV, as it is more cost-effective.
10. Store unopened vials of insulin in the refrigerator; a vial currently in use can be stored at room temperature for up to 1 month and should be kept out of direct sunlight.
11. Prefilled syringes should be stored vertically with the needle pointing up to avoid clogging the needle; gently agitate the syringe to resuspend the insulin before use. May be stored in refrigerator for at least 1 week, perhaps 2 weeks.

ORAL ANTIDIABETIC DRUGS & NONINSULIN INJECTABLE AGENTS

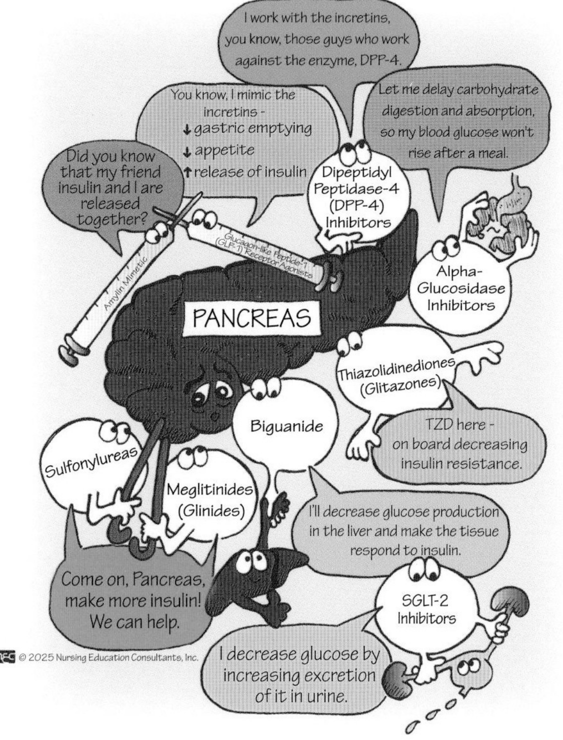

What You Need to Know

Oral Antidiabetic Drugs and Noninsulin Injectable Agents

TYPES

- Oral antidiabetic drugs
  - Seven types are available: the biguanides, sulfonylureas, meglitinides (glinides), thiazolidinediones (glitazones or TZDs), alpha-glucosidase inhibitors, dipeptidyl peptidase-4 (DPP-4) inhibitors (gliptins), and sodium-glucose cotransporter 2 (SGLT-2) inhibitors. Used for type 2 diabetes
- Noninsulin injectable agents
  - Glucagon-like peptide-1 receptor agonists: exenatide (Byetta), liraglutide (Victoza), lixisenatide (Adlyxin), and dulaglutide (Trulicity)
    - Indicated for only type 2 diabetes
  - Amylin mimetic: pramlintide (Symlin)
    - Can be used for type 1 and type 2 diabetes

ACTIONS ■ Black Box Warning

- Sulfonylureas and meglitinides (glinides), collectively referred to as "insulin secretagogues," decrease blood glucose by increasing insulin release from beta cells of the pancreas.
- Metformin (a biguanide), the alpha-glucosidase inhibitors, and SGLT-2 inhibitors do not actively decrease blood glucose, but simply modulate the rise in glucose that happens after a meal.
  - Metformin (a biguanide) decreases glucose production by the liver, increases glucose uptake by the muscle and adipose tissue, and decreases absorption of glucose in the gut.
  - Alpha-glucosidase inhibitors (acarbose, miglitol) act in the intestine to delay digestion and absorption of carbohydrates.
  - SGLT-2 inhibitors (flozins or gliflozins) block the reabsorption of filtered glucose in the kidney, leading to increased urinary glucose excretion.
- TZDs (glitazones) reduce insulin resistance by increasing glucose uptake by the muscle and adipose tissue and decreasing glucose production by the liver; two medications are available, pioglitazone (Actos) and rosiglitazone (Avandia).
- DPP-4 inhibitors (gliptins) enhance the action of the incretin hormones, which stimulate glucose-dependent release of insulin and suppress postprandial release of glucagon (decreases glucose production by the liver).

SULFONYLUREAS

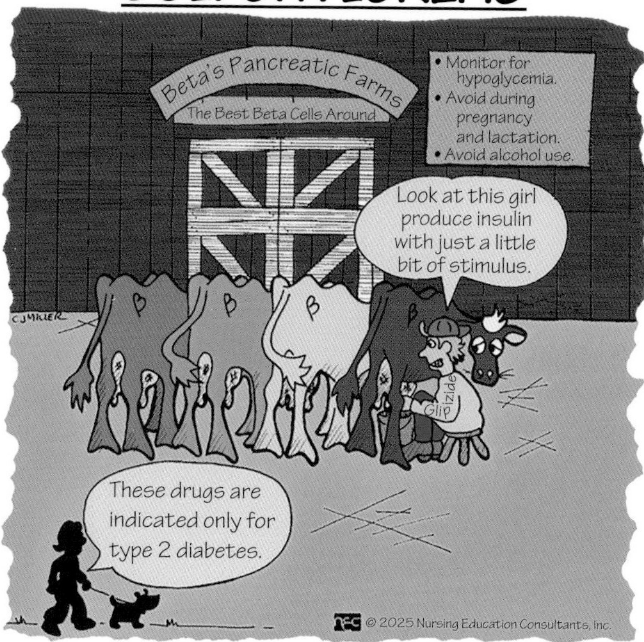

What You Need to Know

Sulfonylureas

- First generation—all have been discontinued in the United States
- Second generation—glipizide (Glucotrol), glyburide (Glynase), glimepiride (Amaryl)

ACTIONS ▲ High Alert

Stimulates the beta cells of the pancreas to increase release of insulin. May also increase cellular sensitivity to insulin. Second-generation medications act the same but are stronger and have fewer drug-drug interactions.

USES

- Type 2 diabetes
- Used as adjunct to diet and exercise to maintain glucose control

CONTRAINDICATIONS AND PRECAUTIONS

- Pregnancy and breast-feeding
- Not effective in patients with type 1 diabetes
- Use with caution in patients with adrenal or pituitary insufficiency or severe hepatic or kidney impairment

SIDE EFFECTS

- Hypoglycemia and weight gain

NURSING IMPLICATIONS

1. Instruct patient to take with food if gastrointestinal upset occurs; otherwise, take the drug 15 to 30 minutes before meals. Do not take medication and skip meals.
2. Self-monitor blood glucose levels as directed.
3. Teach patient to maintain weight and dietary restrictions along with medication; avoid alcohol.
4. Hypoglycemia (fatigue, hunger, tachycardia, sweating, headache, confusion, dizziness, palpitations) should be treated immediately—take fast-acting oral carbohydrates (e.g., glucose tablets, apple juice).
5. Teach family if patient is not in the hospital and cannot swallow or is unresponsive, emergency services (9-1-1) should be initiated.

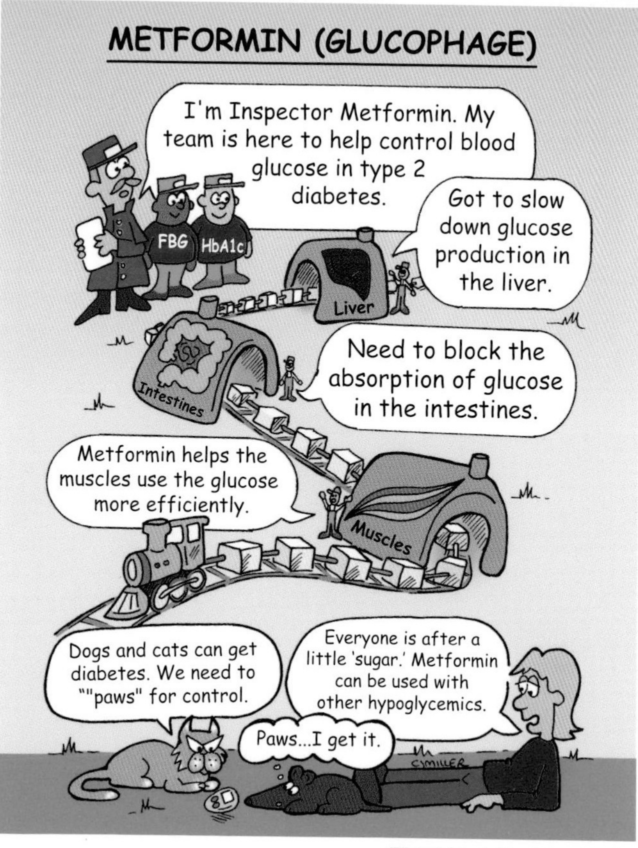
METFORMIN (GLUCOPHAGE)
I'm Inspector Metformin. My team is here to help control blood glucose in type 2 diabetes.
FBG
HbA1c
Got to slow down glucose production in the liver.
Liver
Need to block the absorption of glucose in the intestines.
Intestines
Metformin helps the muscles use the glucose more efficiently.
Muscles
Dogs and cats can get diabetes. We need to ""paws" for control.
Everyone is after a little 'sugar.' Metformin can be used with other hypoglycemics.
Paws...I get it.
C.MILLER

What You Need to Know

Metformin (Glucophage)

CLASSIFICATION

Oral antidiabetic ■ Black Box Warning ▲ High Alert

ACTIONS

Lowers blood glucose and improves glucose tolerance by inhibiting glucose production in the liver, reducing (slightly) glucose absorption in the gut, and sensitizing insulin receptors at sites in fat and skeletal muscle cells, which increases glucose uptake by fat cells and skeletal muscle cells, thereby lowering blood glucose levels.

USES

- Lowers blood glucose level in patients with type 2 diabetes
- May be used for blood glucose level control in patients with gestational diabetes
- Off-label use—polycystic ovary syndrome (PCOS)

CONTRAINDICATIONS

- Conditions that predispose a patient to lactic acidosis (e.g., liver disease, severe infections, hypoxemia, dehydration), severe kidney dysfunction

PRECAUTIONS

- Patients who consume large amounts of alcohol
- Heart failure may predispose patient to lactic acidosis
- Patients with kidney failure

SIDE EFFECTS

- Decreased appetite, nausea, diarrhea, abdominal cramping
- Decreased absorption of vitamin B_{12} and folic acid
- Lactic acidosis

NURSING IMPLICATIONS

1. Monitor serum glucose and HbA1c levels.
2. Assess effectiveness of blood glucose level control when used with other oral hypoglycemics (sulfonylureas).
3. Teach patient to:
   - Avoid alcohol.
   - Take medication as scheduled (do not skip or add doses; do not stop taking medication).
   - Maintain dietary restrictions for glucose control.
4. Teach patient the signs of lactic acidosis: hyperventilation, muscle aches, extreme fatigue.
5. Encourage patient to increase vitamin B12 and folic acid in diet.

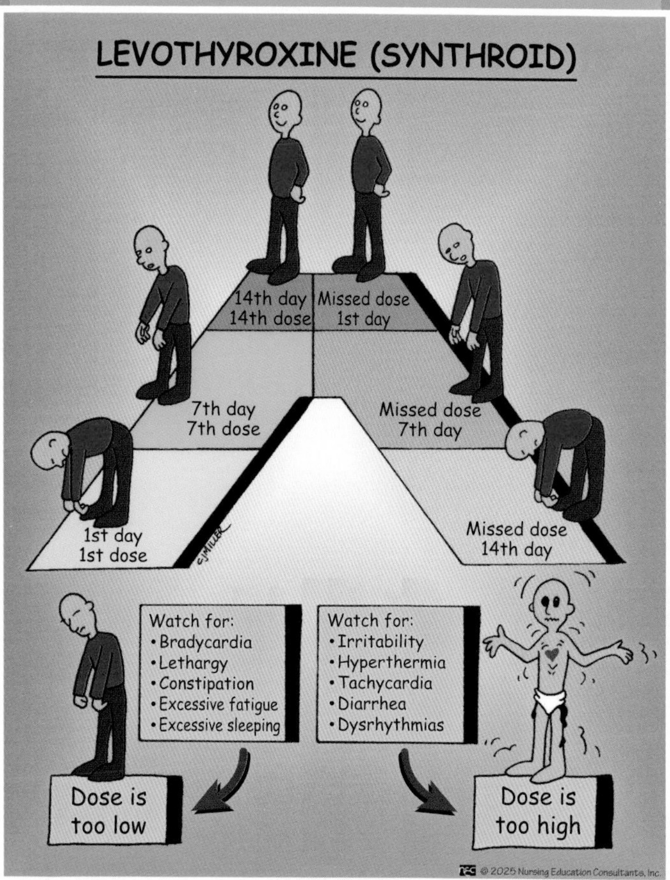
LEVOTHYROXINE (SYNTHROID)
14th day
14th dose
Missed dose
1st day
7th day
7th dose
Missed dose
7th day
1st day
1st dose
Missed dose
14th day
CJMILLER
Watch for:
• Bradycardia
• Lethargy
• Constipation
• Excessive fatigue
• Excessive sleeping
Watch for:
• Irritability
• Hyperthermia
• Tachycardia
• Diarrhea
• Dysrhythmias
Dose is
too low
Dose is
too high
© 2025 Nursing Education Consultants, Inc.

What You Need to Know

Levothyroxine (Synthroid)

CLASSIFICATION

Thyroid hormone; synthetic preparation of thyroxine

ACTIONS ■ Black Box Warning

Increases basal metabolic rate, enhances gluconeogenesis, stimulates protein synthesis

USES

- Replacement in decreased or absent thyroid function
- Hypothyroidism, cretinism, myxedema coma, simple goiter
- Management of thyroid cancer following surgery

CONTRAINDICATIONS AND PRECAUTIONS

- Thyrotoxicosis and myocardial infarction without hypothyroidism
- Treatment of obesity
- Older adult patients, patients with impaired cardiac function, hypertension

SIDE EFFECTS

- Overdose may cause thyrotoxicosis—tachycardia, increased blood pressure, angina, tremor, nervousness, insomnia, heat intolerance, hyperthermia, sweating
- Long-term use—osteoporosis and increased risk for atrial fibrillation

NURSING IMPLICATIONS

1. Monitor for tachycardia and irregular pulse rate.
2. Teach patient to report any symptoms of thyrotoxicosis.
3. Replacement for hypothyroidism is lifelong. Do not discontinue medication.
4. Instruct patient to have thyroid-stimulating hormone levels measured periodically.
5. Takes approximately 6 to 8 weeks for the full effects of the medication to be seen.
6. Teach patient to take the medication in the morning, preferably 30 to 60 minutes before meals.
7. Advise patient to take 4 hours apart from antacids, calcium supplements, and iron preparations.

AGE-RELATED MACULAR DEGENERATION (ARMD)

Ranibizumab (Lucentis), Aflibercept (Eylea), Bevacizumab (Avastin), Pegaptanib (Macugen)

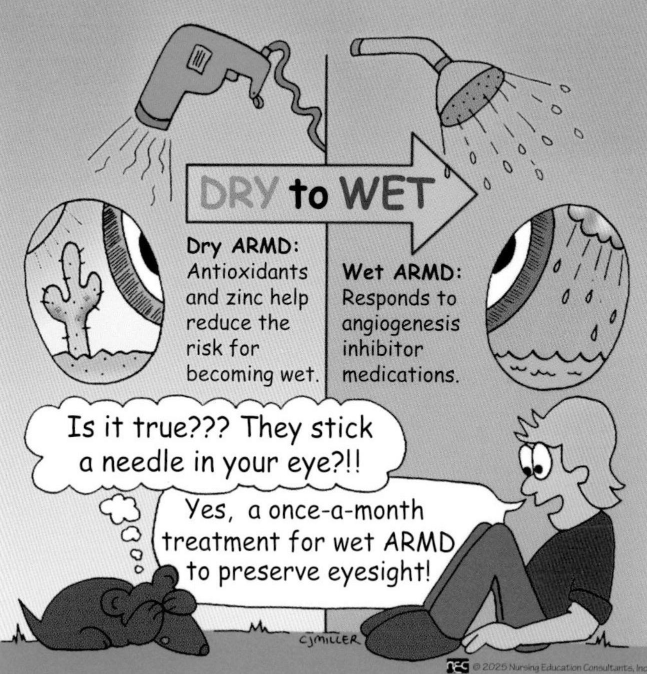

What You Need to Know

Drugs for Age-Related Macular Degeneration

CLASSIFICATION

Angiogenesis inhibitor

Four drugs: ranibizumab (Lucentis), aflibercept (Eylea), bevacizumab (Avastin), pegaptanib (Macugen)

ACTIONS

Note: Some medications are ■ **Black Box Warning** and ▲ **High Alert**

Drug works by antagonizing vascular endothelial growth factor (VEGF). VEGF causes angiogenesis (growth of new retinal vessels that are fragile and leaky), increases vascular permeability, and promotes inflammation contributing to wet age-related macular degeneration (ARMD).

TWO TYPES OF ARMD

- Dry ARMD (atrophic)—more common; less severe
- Wet ARMD (neovascular)—less common; more severe

  Disorder begins as dry ARMD and can progress to wet ARMD.

TREATMENT

- Dry ARMD (atrophic)
  - High doses of antioxidants (vitamins C and E, beta-carotene) and zinc
- Wet ARMD (neovascular)
  - **Laser therapy**—seals leaky blood vessels
  - **Photodynamic therapy**—uses a photosensitive drug in combination with infrared light to seal leaky blood vessels
  - **Angiogenesis inhibitors**—preferred treatment compared with laser and photodynamic therapy; pegaptanib (Macugen) is used rarely

SIDE EFFECTS

- Endophthalmitis—inflammation inside the eye caused by bacterial, viral, or fungal infection; redness, light sensitivity
- Blurred vision, cataracts, ocular discomfort, corneal edema, eye discharge, conjunctival hemorrhage

NURSING IMPLICATIONS

1. Teach patient with dry ARMD the importance of a preventive diet of antioxidants and zinc.
2. Monitor for copper-induced anemia caused by high doses of zinc; may need to supplement with copper as prescribed.
3. Intravitreal injection (directly into the vitreous of the eye) of angiogenesis inhibitors usually monthly.

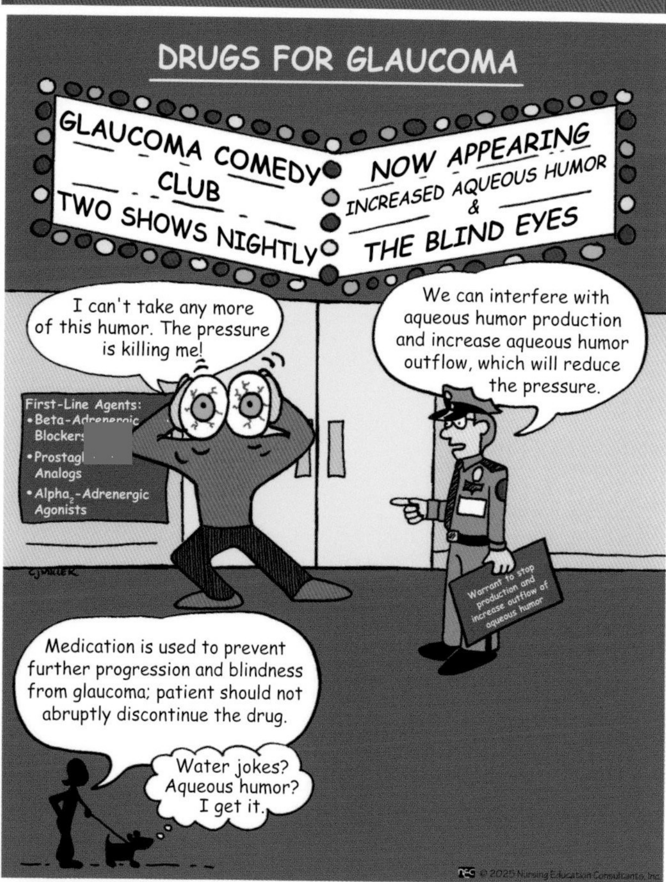

DRUGS FOR GLAUCOMA
GLAUCOMA COMEDY CLUB
TWO SHOWS NIGHTLY
NOW APPEARING
INCREASED AQUEOUS HUMOR
&
THE BLIND EYES
I can't take any more of this humor. The pressure is killing me!
We can interfere with aqueous humor production and increase aqueous humor outflow, which will reduce the pressure.
First-Line Agents:
• Beta-Adrenergic Blockers
• Prostagl Analogs
• Alpha2-Adrenergic Agonists
Warrant to stop production and increase outflow of aqueous humor
Medication is used to prevent further progression and blindness from glaucoma; patient should not abruptly discontinue the drug.
Water jokes? Aqueous humor? I get it.

What You Need to Know

Drugs for Glaucoma

EXAMPLES

Beta-adrenergic blocking agents or *Beta-blockers:* timolol (Timoptic); blocks $beta_1$- and $beta_2$-receptors; betaxolol (Betoptic): $beta_1$-selective
Prostaglandin analogs: latanoprost (Xalatan)
Alpha-adrenergic agonists: brimonidine (Alphagan)

ACTIONS

Beta-blockers: reduce production of aqueous humor and thereby promote a decrease in intraocular pressure. When systemically absorbed, blockage of $beta_1$-receptors may cause bradycardia and heart block; blockage of $beta_2$-receptors in the lung may cause bronchospasm.
Prostaglandin analogs: increase aqueous humor outflow.
Alpha-adrenergic agonists: reduce aqueous humor production.

USES

- Primary open-angle glaucoma; ocular hypertension

CONTRAINDICATIONS

- Severe bradycardia, atrioventricular heart block, cardiogenic shock (beta-blockers)

PRECAUTIONS

- Heart failure, hypotension, asthma, chronic obstructive pulmonary disease (COPD)

SIDE EFFECTS

- Beta-blockers: decreased visual acuity, ocular burning, conjunctivitis, photophobia, bradycardia and pulmonary implications (bronchospasm) if absorbed systemically
- Latanoprost: brown pigmentation of iris/eyelids; increases eyelash growth
- Brimonidine: dry mouth, headache, altered taste, drowsiness, hypotension

NURSING IMPLICATIONS

1. Assess patient for systemic absorption of medication (bradycardia, hypotension).
2. Teach patient to apply slight pressure at the inner canthus for 1 minute after instillation to decrease systemic absorption of medication.
3. Teach patient about spacing out eye drops by 5 to 15 minutes if multiple ones need to be instilled in the same eye to prevent dilution.
4. Wait 15 minutes after eye drop instillation before applying contact lenses.

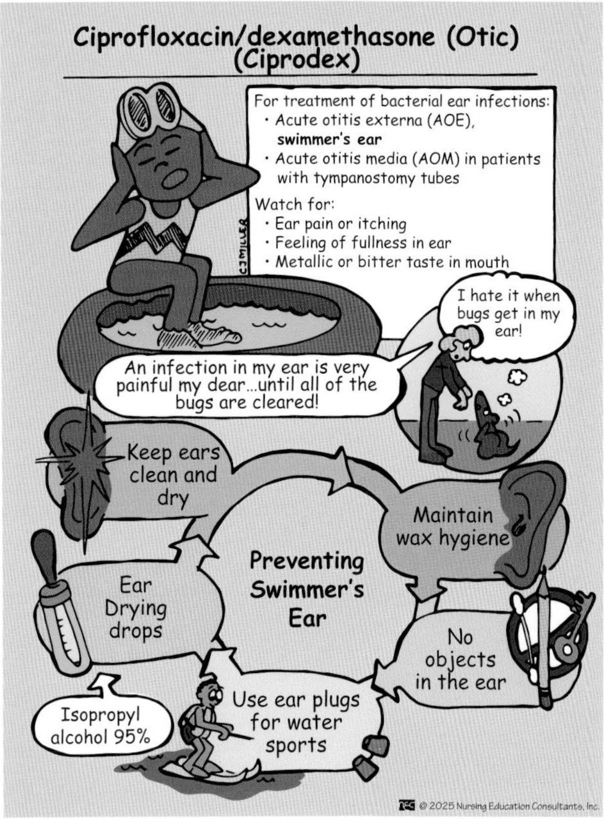

Ciprofloxacin/dexamethasone (Otic) (Ciprodex)

For treatment of bacterial ear infections:

- Acute otitis externa (AOE), **swimmer's ear**
- Acute otitis media (AOM) in patients with tympanostomy tubes

Watch for:

- Ear pain or itching
- Feeling of fullness in ear
- Metallic or bitter taste in mouth

CJ MILLER

I hate it when bugs get in my ear!

An infection in my ear is very painful my dear...until all of the bugs are cleared!

Preventing Swimmer's Ear

Keep ears clean and dry

Maintain wax hygiene

No objects in the ear

Use ear plugs for water sports

Ear Drying drops

Isopropyl alcohol 95%

What You Need to Know

Ciprofloxacin/Dexamethasone (Ciprodex)

CLASSIFICATION

Fluoroquinolone/corticosteroid

ACTIONS

Antimicrobial agent stops microbial growth of pathogen and the corticosteroid reduces inflammation and pain associated with the bacterial ear infection.

USES

- Acute otitis externa; swimmer's ear
- Acute otitis media in patients with tympanostomy tubes

CONTRAINDICATIONS

- Hypersensitivity to ciprofloxacin or fluoroquinolones
- Viral infections of the ear

PRECAUTIONS

- For otic (ear) use only
- Potential for microbial overgrowth with prolonged use
- Prolonged use can promote resistance to fluoroquinolone antibiotics

SIDE EFFECTS

- Altered taste, ear pruritus, ear pain/discomfort, ear precipitate, angioedema

NURSING IMPLICATIONS

1. Teach patient and family to warm bottle in their hand for 1 minute and shake well right before administration.
2. Protect medication from light.
3. Teach patient and family measures for preventing recurrent bacterial ear infections (keep ears dry, do not place objects in ears, do not remove cerumen from ears, and use ear plugs for watersports and swimming).
4. Advise patient and family to continue using eardrops as prescribed, even if symptoms improve.

H_2-Receptor Antagonists (H_2RAs)

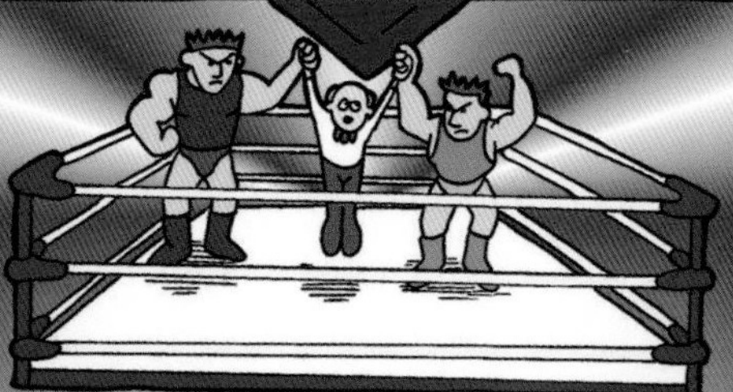

What You Need to Know

H_2-Receptor Antagonists

TYPES

Cimetidine (Tagamet), famotidine (Pepcid). (*Note the "tidine" ending in the generic names.*)

ACTION

H_2-receptor antagonists (H_2RAs) inhibit histamine action on H_2 receptors, which are found on the gastric parietal cells. This action reduces the secretion of gastric acid as well as hydrogen ion concentration.

USES

- Prevention and treatment of gastric and duodenal ulcers
- Heartburn, acid indigestion, and gastroesophageal reflux disease (GERD)

CONTRAINDICATIONS AND PRECAUTIONS

- Caution with hepatic and kidney dysfunction
- Caution in older adult patients
- Antacids can decrease absorption, especially with cimetidine

SIDE EFFECTS

- Diarrhea, constipation
- Older adults: confusion, agitation
- Decrease in stomach acid may increase growth of *Candida* and bacteria in stomach, resulting in increased risk for pneumonia
- Cimetidine: May bind with androgens to cause gynecomastia and impotence; effects reverse after medication is withdrawn; may cause hypotension and dysrhythmias when given as intravenous bolus

NURSING IMPLICATIONS

1. Oral medications may be taken without regard to meals.
2. At least 1 hour should separate the administration of antacids and cimetidine.
3. Teach patient to avoid alcohol.
4. Smoking increases gastric acid secretion, which may decrease effectiveness.
5. Teach patient the signs of gastric bleeding (black tarry stools, "coffee-ground" emesis) and to notify health care provider (HCP) if any occur.
6. Teach patient to notify HCP for any indication of respiratory problems.
7. Teach patient that five to six small meals a day may be preferable to three large meals a day.

PSYLLIUM (METAMUCIL)

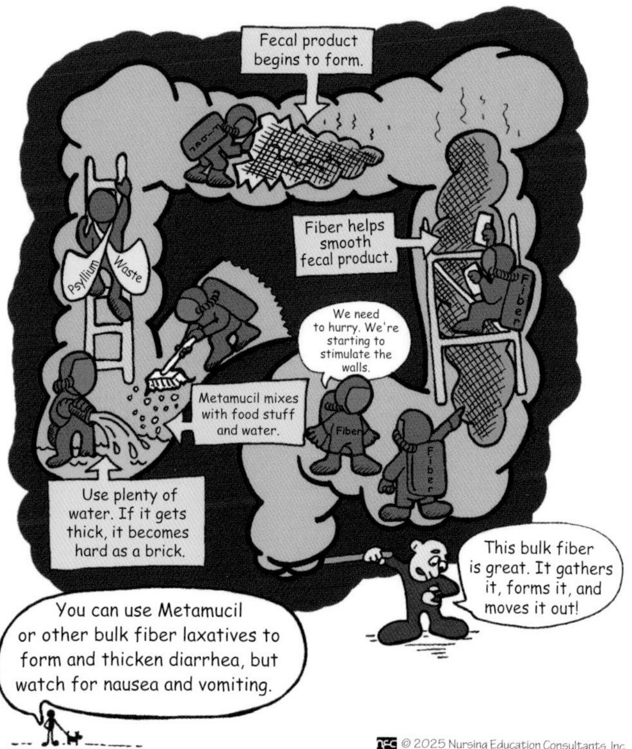

What You Need to Know

Psyllium (Metamucil)

CLASSIFICATION

Bulk-forming laxative

ACTIONS

Acts similar to dietary fiber. This medication is not digested or absorbed. After ingestion, it will swell to form a viscous solution or gel, softening the fecal mass and increasing the bulk. A fecal mass stretches the intestinal wall to stimulate peristalsis and passage of a soft-formed stool in 1 to 3 days.

USES

- Treats constipation; preferred agent for temporary treatment of constipation
- Diverticulosis and irritable bowel syndrome
- Relief of diarrhea for patients with an ileostomy or colostomy

CONTRAINDICATIONS

- Fecal impaction or any condition leading to narrowing of the intestinal lumen
- Bowel obstruction or undiagnosed acute abdominal pain

PRECAUTIONS

- Esophageal obstruction can occur if medication is swallowed without sufficient fluid
- Intestinal adhesions, ulcers, narrowing of intestinal lumen

SIDE EFFECTS

- Abdominal discomfort, bloating
- Impaction and intestinal obstruction if not given with adequate liquids

NURSING IMPLICATIONS

1. Mix medication with at least 8 ounces of water; mix at the bedside immediately before administration.
2. Instruct patient to drink at least 8 ounces of water after each dose and drink at least six to eight glasses of water each day to facilitate peristalsis and to prevent obstruction.
3. Bowel movement should occur in 1 to 3 days.
4. Administer at least 2 hours before or after medications.

Important nursing implications | Serious/life-threatening implications

Most frequent side effects | Patient teaching

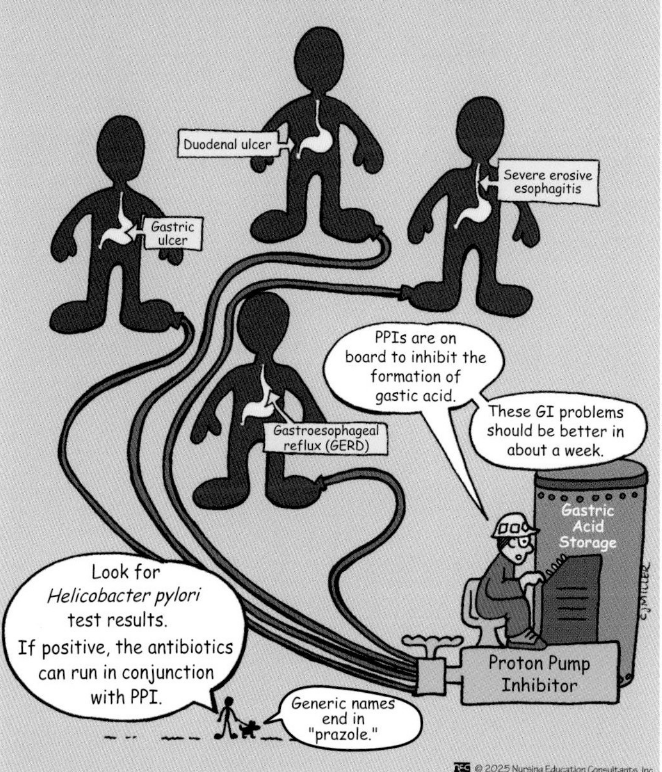
PROTON PUMP INHIBITORS (PPIs)
Duodenal ulcer
Severe erosive esophagitis
Gastric ulcer
PPIs are on board to inhibit the formation of gastic acid.
These GI problems should be better in about a week.
Gastroesophageal reflux (GERD)
Gastric Acid Storage
Look for *Helicobacter pylori* test results. If positive, the antibiotics can run in conjunction with PPI.
Proton Pump Inhibitor
Generic names end in "prazole."
© 2025 Nursing Education Consultants, Inc.

What You Need to Know

Proton Pump Inhibitors

EXAMPLES

Omeprazole (Prilosec), esomeprazole (Nexium), lansoprazole (Prevacid), pantoprazole (Protonix). (*Note the "prazole" ending in all the generic names.*)

ACTIONS

Most effective drug in suppressing the secretion of gastric acid by combining with an enzyme on the gastric parietal cells; block the final common pathway for gastric acid formation; decrease hydrogen ion transport into the gastric lumen.

USES

- Short term (4–8 weeks): duodenal ulcers associated with *Helicobacter pylori*, gastric ulcers, erosive gastritis, and GERD
- Long term: hypersecretory conditions (Zollinger-Ellison syndrome)
- Stress ulcer prophylaxis for patients in intensive care settings

CONTRAINDICATIONS AND PRECAUTIONS

- Long-term use may predispose patient to the risk of developing *Clostridioides difficile* and gastrointestinal (GI) infections (e.g., salmonella), especially in hospitalized patients
- Long-term therapy may predispose patient to the risk of osteoporosis and fractures
- Use with caution in hepatic impairment

SIDE EFFECTS

- Headache, diarrhea, nausea, vomiting
- Long-term therapy: pneumonia, fractures, rebound acid hypersecretion, hypomagnesemia, vitamin B_{12} deficiency

NURSING IMPLICATIONS

1. Instruct patient to avoid opening, splitting, chewing, or crushing capsules and tablets.
2. Instruct patient to return for follow-up if symptoms are unresolved after 4 to 8 weeks of therapy.
3. Teach patient to take medication before meals.
4. Encourage patient to maintain adequate intake of calcium, magnesium, vitamin D.
5. Teach patient to report any symptoms of hypomagnesemia (tremor, muscle cramps, seizures, dysrhythmias).
6. Teach patient to report any symptoms of respiratory infection (dyspnea, fever, productive cough).

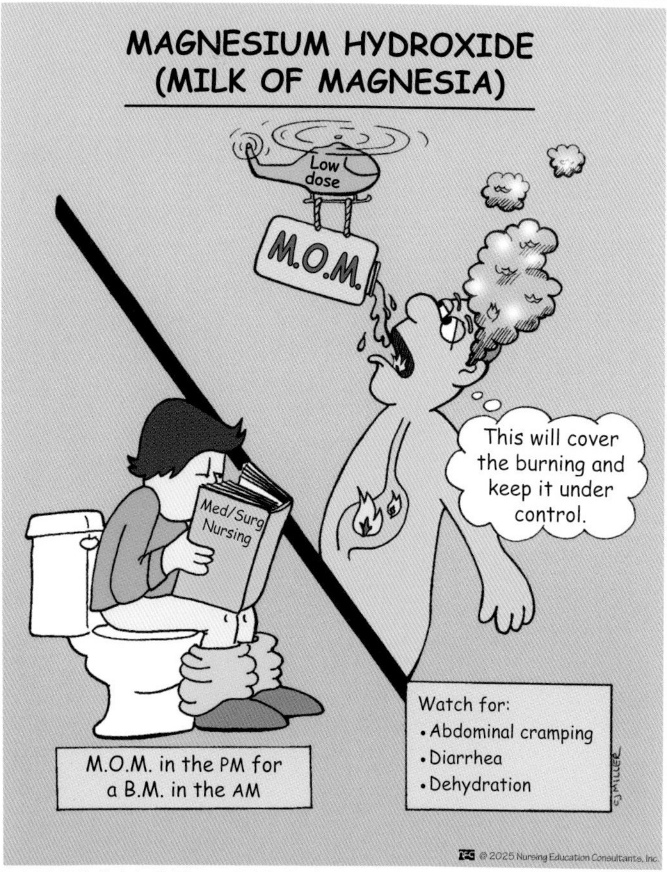

MAGNESIUM HYDROXIDE (MILK OF MAGNESIA)

Low dose

M.O.M.

This will cover the burning and keep it under control.

Med/Surg Nursing

M.O.M. in the PM for a B.M. in the AM

Watch for:
- Abdominal cramping
- Diarrhea
- Dehydration

CJ MILLER

What You Need to Know

Magnesium Hydroxide (Milk of Magnesia)

CLASSIFICATION

Osmotic laxative, magnesium compound (antacid)

ACTIONS

Draws water into the intestine by osmotic action on the surrounding tissue. The increase in fluid in the intestine will cause the stool to expand and soften. This causes stretching of the bowel and increases peristalsis. Rapid-acting antacid with high acid-neutralizing capacity and long-lasting effects.

USES

- Constipation
- Bowel prep for diagnostic procedure or surgery
- Flush ingested toxins out of the GI tract
- Antacid

CONTRAINDICATIONS

- Undiagnosed abdominal pain
- Kidney impairment

PRECAUTIONS

- Rectal bleeding
- Bowel obstructions
- Colostomy or ileostomy

SIDE EFFECTS

- Abdominal cramping, diarrhea, dehydration
- Hypermagnesemia—magnesium toxicity (central nervous system depression) can occur in patient with kidney impairment

NURSING IMPLICATIONS

1. Give with at least 8 ounces of water.
2. Will generally act within 6 to 12 hours.
3. Monitor bowel movement, hydration status, and electrolyte levels.
4. Laxative abuse (laxative taken every day) decreases the defecation reflex, leading to laxative dependence.
5. Teach patient to eat foods high in fiber (brans, fruits) and increase fluid intake.
6. For antacid use, it is commonly given with aluminum hydroxide to alleviate common symptoms of diarrhea.

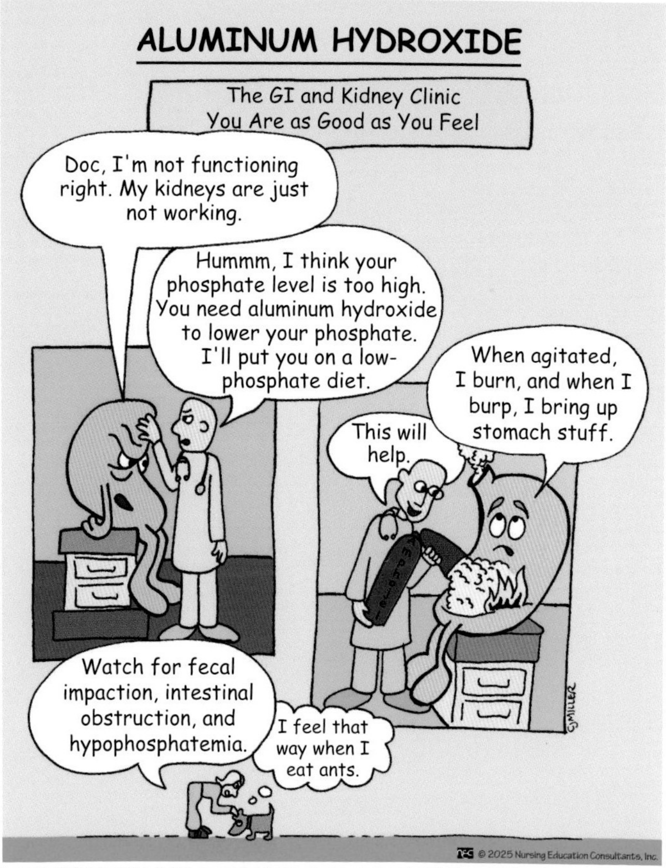

ALUMINUM HYDROXIDE

The GI and Kidney Clinic
You Are as Good as You Feel

Doc, I'm not functioning right. My kidneys are just not working.

Hummm, I think your phosphate level is too high. You need aluminum hydroxide to lower your phosphate. I'll put you on a low-phosphate diet.

When agitated, I burn, and when I burp, I bring up stomach stuff.

This will help.

Watch for fecal impaction, intestinal obstruction, and hypophosphatemia.

I feel that way when I eat ants.

What You Need to Know

Aluminum Hydroxide

CLASSIFICATION

Phosphate-binding antacid, aluminum compound

ACTIONS

Reduces acid concentration and pepsin activity by raising pH of gastric secretions. Binds with phosphate and helps prevent hyperphosphatemia. Decrease in serum phosphorous level may precipitate an increase in serum calcium level.

USES

- Relieves hyperacidity related to gastritis and reflux
- Treats gastric and duodenal ulcers
- May be used to treat hyperphosphatemia in renal insufficiency
- Most frequently used in combination with magnesium hydroxide

CONTRAINDICATIONS AND PRECAUTIONS

- Dehydration or fluid restriction or both
- Renal disease or cardiac disease or both
- Undiagnosed abdominal pain, intestinal obstruction, chronic constipation, diarrhea
- Binds to tetracyclines, warfarin, digoxin and may reduce their effect

SIDE EFFECTS

- Constipation, abdominal cramps, hypophosphatemia

NURSING IMPLICATIONS

1. Monitor serum calcium, phosphate, magnesium, sodium levels.
2. Do not administer antacids to patients with a cardiac presentation who complain of dyspepsia; discomfort may be referred anginal pain.
3. Teach patient to shake suspensions thoroughly before use and to thoroughly chew tablets before swallowing.
4. Administer at least 2 hours before or after medications.
5. Teach patient to take medication before meals, when stomach acidity is highest.

Important nursing implications | Serious/life-threatening implications
Most frequent side effects | Patient teaching

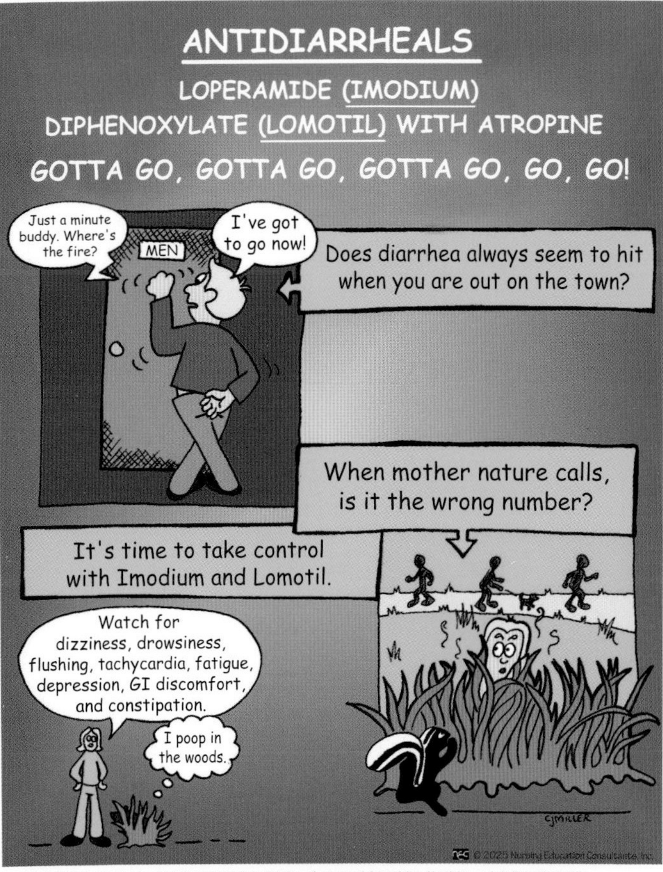
ANTIDIARRHEALS
LOPERAMIDE (IMODIUM)
DIPHENOXYLATE (LOMOTIL) WITH ATROPINE
GOTTA GO, GOTTA GO, GOTTA GO, GO, GO!
Just a minute buddy. Where's the fire?
MEN
I've got to go now!
Does diarrhea always seem to hit when you are out on the town?
When mother nature calls, is it the wrong number?
It's time to take control with Imodium and Lomotil.
Watch for dizziness, drowsiness, flushing, tachycardia, fatigue, depression, GI discomfort, and constipation.
I poop in the woods.
CJMILLER
© 2025 Nursing Education Consultants, Inc.

What You Need to Know

Antidiarrheals

EXAMPLES

Loperamide (Imodium), diphenoxylate with atropine (Lomotil)

ACTIONS

Direct effect on intestinal motility; slows intestinal transit and allows for increased absorption of fluids and electrolytes. Diphenoxylate is an opioid (Schedule V) and is combined with atropine to discourage the abuse of taking high doses to experience opioid euphoria. Loperamide is an analog of meperidine and has little or no potential for abuse.

USES

- Symptomatic relief of acute nonspecific diarrhea
- Chronic diarrhea associated with inflammatory bowel disease
- Reduces high-stoma output associated with ileostomies

CONTRAINDICATIONS AND PRECAUTIONS

- Hepatic or kidney disease (loperamide)
- Dehydration with electrolyte depletion
- Diarrhea from colitis or from infectious organism (slowing peristalsis may delay the removal of the infecting organism, which may prolong the infection)
- Loperamide and diphenoxylate with atropine are not used in children younger than 2 years of age
- Undiagnosed abdominal pain

SIDE EFFECTS

- Drowsiness, dizziness, abdominal discomfort

NURSING IMPLICATIONS

1. Encourage adequate fluid intake; monitor hydration status.
2. Check bowel sounds for peristalsis; discontinue and report abdominal pain and distention.
3. Do not give in the presence of bloody diarrhea or a temperature of greater than 101°F (38.3°C).
4. Avoid alcohol (diphenoxylate with atropine).

Important nursing implications | Serious/life-threatening implications
Most frequent side effects | Patient teaching

LACTULOSE

You have portal hypertension. Your liver is not working right. Here is some lactulose to help flush out the ammonia in your intestinal tract. Lactulose also works as a strong osmotic laxative.

LACTULOSE

The side effects are belching, abdominal distention, flatulence, nausea and vomiting, and diarrhea.

Check your ammonia labs.

CJ MILLER

What You Need to Know

Lactulose

CLASSIFICATION

Hyperosmotic laxative and ammonia detoxicant

ACTIONS

Pulls ammonia into the colon from the intestines; promotes increased peristalsis, bowel evacuation (expelling ammonia from colon); decreases serum ammonia concentration in the body.

USES

- Treats portal systemic (hepatic) encephalopathy
- Treats constipation unresponsive to bulk laxatives

CONTRAINDICATIONS

- Undiagnosed abdominal pain, nausea, vomiting

PRECAUTIONS

- Diabetes mellitus
- Dehydration

SIDE EFFECTS

- Abdominal cramping, flatulence, bloating, nausea, vomiting.
- Frequent loose stools may be desirable in excretion of ammonia; may be a side effect if used for constipation.

NURSING IMPLICATIONS

1. Encourage increased fluid intake and high-fiber diet.
2. Monitor bowel activity; may receive dose even with loose stools.
3. Monitor serum ammonia and electrolyte levels.
4. Do not use with other laxatives (hepatic encephalopathy).
5. May be given by mouth (PO) or by enema:
   - PO: Mix with fruit juice, water, or milk to improve flavor. Take on an empty stomach for rapid action.
   - Rectally: Use rectal balloon catheter; patient needs to retain enema for 30 to 60 minutes. If enema is accidentally expelled, it may be repeated.
6. Teach patient that bowel movement occurs within 1 to 3 days of initial dose.

Important nursing implications | Serious/life-threatening implications

Most frequent side effects | Patient teaching

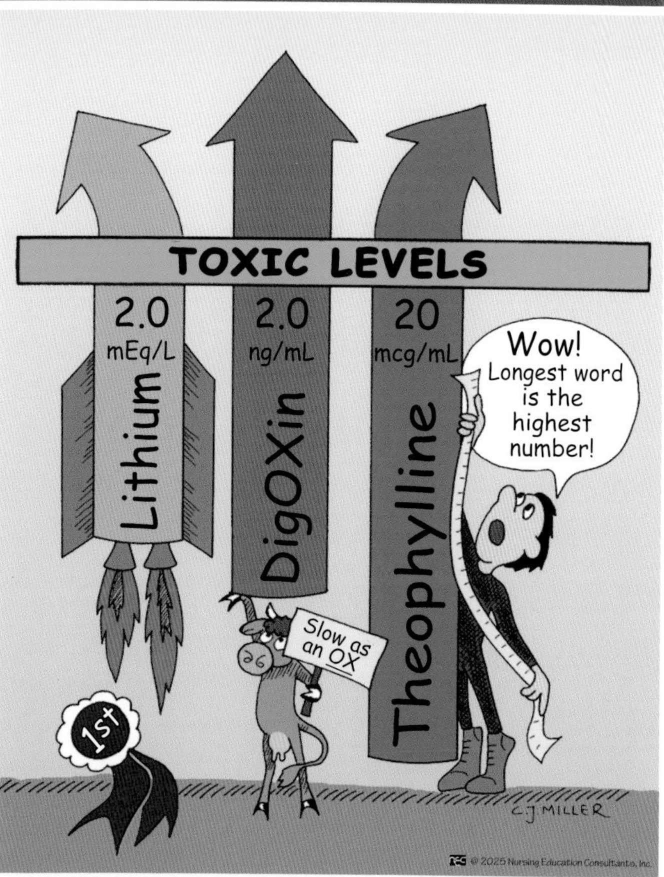
TOXIC LEVELS
2.0
mEq/L
Lithium
2.0
ng/mL
DigOXin
20
mcg/mL
Theophylline
Wow!
Longest word
is the
highest
number!
Slow as
an OX
1st
C.J. MILLER
© 2025 Nursing Education Consultants, Inc.

What You Need to Know

Toxic Levels of Lithium, Digoxin, and Theophylline

LITHIUM ■ Black Box Warning

- Desired level: 0.6 to 0.8 mEq/L; range level 0.4 to 1.0 mEq/L.
- Toxic level: greater than 2.0 mEq/L (levels should be kept less than 1.5 mEq/L).
- Levels are routinely monitored every 2 to 3 days initially, then every 3 to 6 months during maintenance therapy.
- Sodium depletion is the most common cause of lithium accumulation.

Signs and Symptoms

- Side effects (at therapeutic levels below 1.5 mEq/L) include fine hand tremors, polyuria, thirst, transient fatigue, muscle weakness, headache, memory impairment
- Gastrointestinal (GI) effects are nausea, diarrhea, anorexia
- Toxic effects (1.5–2.0 mEq/L) include persistent GI problems (vomiting, diarrhea), coarse hand tremors, hyperirritability, poor coordination
- Effects of acute toxicity (greater than 2.0 mEq/L) include ataxia, high output of dilute urine, electrocardiographic changes, tinnitus, blurred vision, severe hypotension, seizures. Symptoms may progress to coma and death

DIGOXIN ▲ High Alert

- Optimal level: 0.5 to 0.8 ng/mL.
- Toxic level: greater than 2.0 ng/mL.
- Hypokalemia is the most common predisposing factor to toxicity.
- Patients should not interchange various brands because of variations in absorption.

Signs and Symptoms

- GI signs include anorexia and nausea and vomiting
- Central nervous system signs are headache, fatigue, and visual disturbances (blurred, yellow-tinge vision; halos around objects)
- Dysrhythmias—digoxin can mimic most dysrhythmias; if cardiac rate or rhythm changes during therapy, the HCP should be notified

THEOPHYLLINE

- Optimal level: 5 to 15 mcg/mL. (*Note: Use of drug has declined sharply.*)
- Toxic level: greater than 20 mcg/mL.
- Signs and symptoms: nausea, vomiting, diarrhea, restlessness (levels 20–25 mcg/mL).

DRUG INTERACTIONS & GRAPEFRUIT

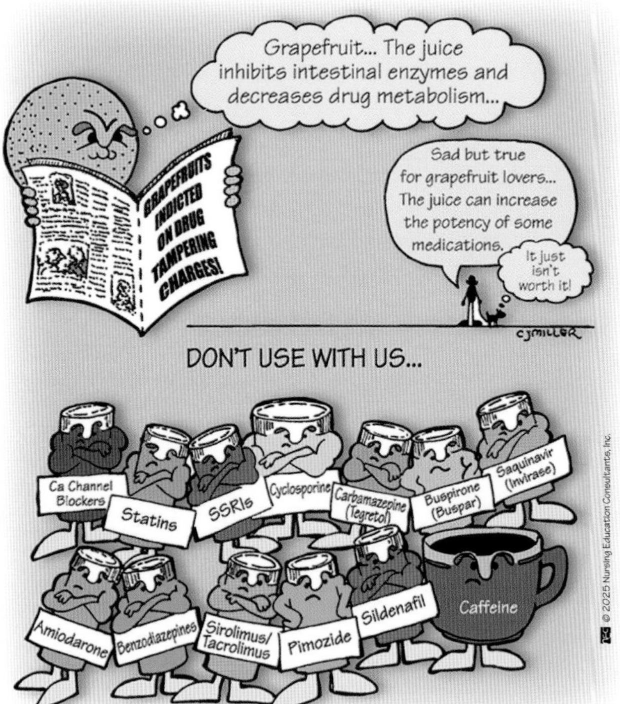

What You Need to Know

Drug Interactions and Grapefruit

CAUTION

Grapefruit inhibits the metabolism of certain drugs, thereby increasing the blood levels of carbamazepine, buspirone, calcium channel blockers (amlodipine, nifedipine, diltiazem, verapamil), benzodiazepines (triazolam, midazolam), statins (lovastatin, simvastatin), cyclosporine, saquinavir, selective serotonin reuptake inhibitors, amiodarone, sirolimus/tacrolimus, pimozide, praziquantel, dextromethorphan, sildenafil, and caffeine.

EFFECT OF GRAPEFRUIT ON MEDICATIONS

- Grapefruit and grapefruit juice are metabolized in the liver by the same enzyme (CYP3A4, an isoenzyme of cytochrome P450) that metabolizes many drugs. When the liver has too many substances to metabolize, the enzymes focus on metabolizing grapefruit while ignoring the medication.
- Because the medication is not being metabolized, it can accumulate to a dangerous level and can lead to intense peak effects.
  - The more grapefruit juice the patient drinks, the greater the inhibition.

NURSING IMPLICATIONS

1. Teach patient to avoid foods and beverages containing grapefruit or grapefruit juice with prescribed drugs whose levels can be increased.
2. Does not affect IV preparations of the medications because intestinal metabolism is not involved.
3. With cyclosporine (Sandimmune) and saquinavir (Invirase), the increased blood level that occurs with consuming grapefruit can intensify the therapeutic effects, which can lead to a good outcome. If levels rise too quickly, nephrotoxicity and hepatotoxicity can occur.

Important nursing implications	Serious/life-threatening implications
Most frequent side effects	Patient teaching

CANCER CHEMOTHERAPY

Adverse Reactions and Precautions

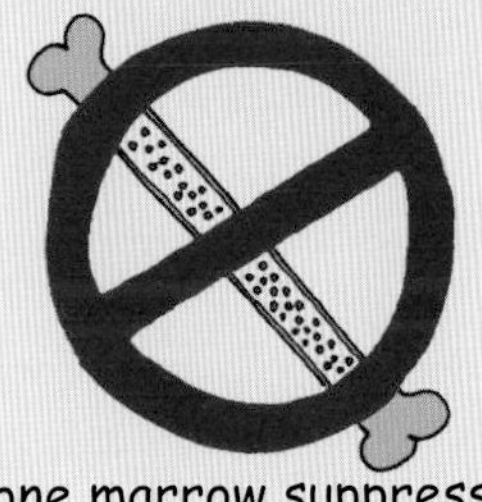

Bone marrow suppression

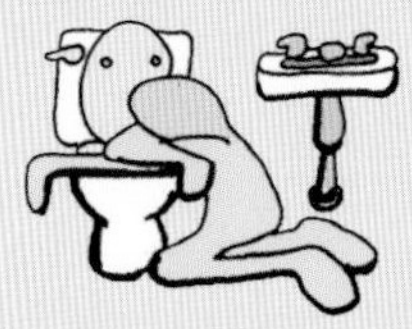

Nausea and vomiting

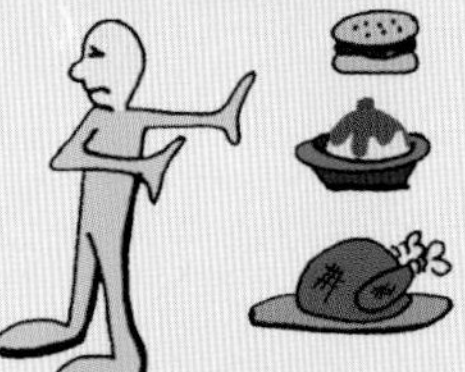

Anorexia

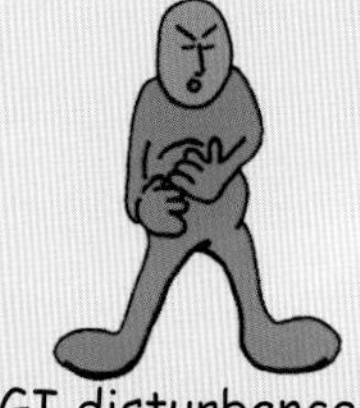

GI disturbances

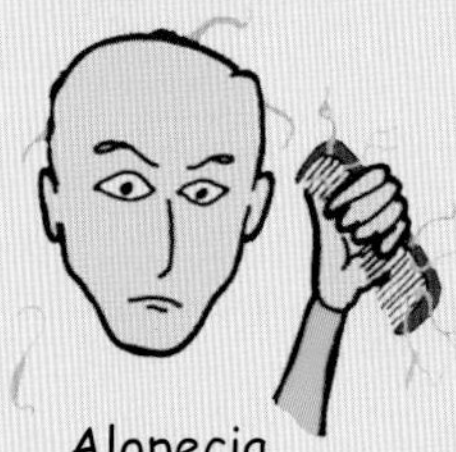

Alopecia

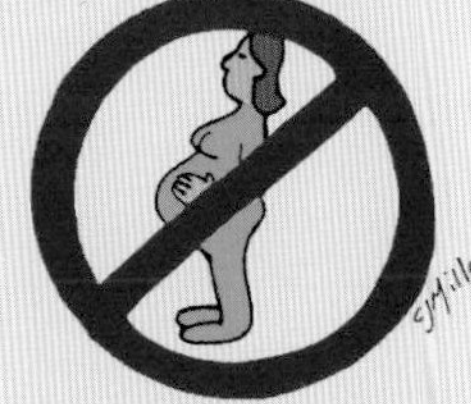

Avoid pregnancy

What You Need to Know

Cancer Chemotherapy: Adverse Reactions and Precautions

ACTIONS ▲ High Alert

Note: All chemotherapy (anticancer) agents are considered high-alert medications; some anticancer agents have a ■ Black Box Warning

Action occurs during the sequence of the cell cycle. Anticancer agents affect cells during any phase of the cell cycle. Other drugs are effective only during a specific phase of the cell cycle. Rapidly dividing cells are more vulnerable to chemotherapy.

DOSAGE, HANDLING, AND ADMINISTRATION

- Medication doses are individualized for each patient.
- Because of the hazardous nature of these medications, it is important that direct contact with the skin, eyes, and mucous membrane is avoided.
- Drugs are frequently given in combination to improve effectiveness of response.

SIDE EFFECTS

- Cytotoxic medications are harmful to normal tissue because they lack selectivity; they kill target cancer cells, but they also kill normal cells.
- Bone marrow suppression: anemia (loss of erythrocytes), thrombocytopenia (bleeding from loss of platelets), and neutropenia (infection from loss of neutrophils) may result.
- GI disturbances: stomatitis (inflammation of oral mucosa), nausea and vomiting, anorexia, diarrhea.
- Alopecia results from injury to hair follicles; regrows 1 to 2 months after treatment.
- Hyperuricemia may cause renal injury secondary to a deposit of urate crystals.
- Reproductive toxicity: fetus is susceptible to injury and malformation.
- Local injury may occur from extravasation of the anticancer drug.

NURSING IMPLICATIONS

1. Monitor for bone marrow suppression; may require an alteration of medication dose.
2. Side effects are expected, and patients are frequently taught how to manage the problems.
3. Observe closely for signs of infection; teach patient to report a fever immediately as this may be the only sign of an infection.
4. Routine laboratory blood tests (complete blood count with differential, blood chemistry panel) are extremely important.

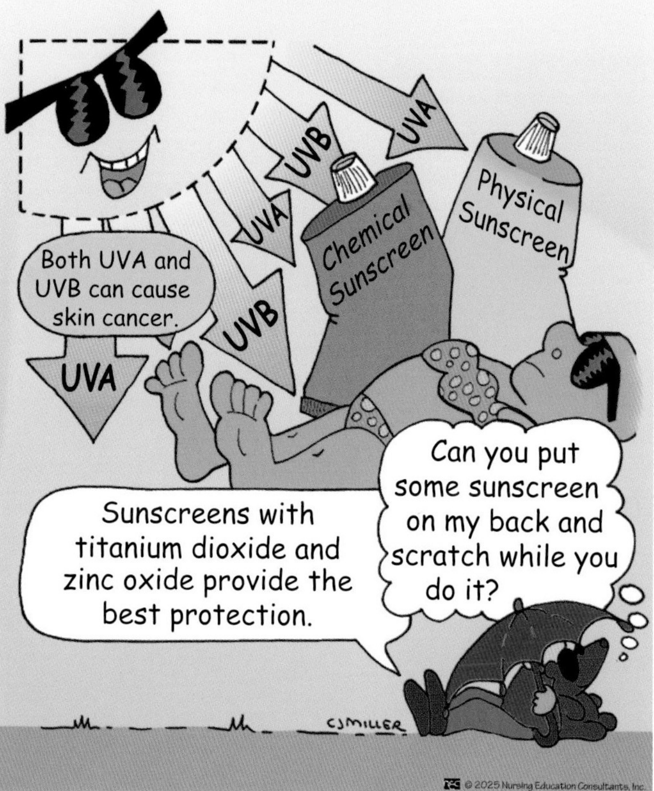
SUNSCREENS
UVB
UVA
UVA
UVB
Both UVA and UVB can cause skin cancer.
UVA
Chemical Sunscreen
Physical Sunscreen
Can you put some sunscreen on my back and scratch while you do it?
Sunscreens with titanium dioxide and zinc oxide provide the best protection.
CJMILLER
© 2025 Nursing Education Consultants, Inc.

What You Need to Know

Sunscreens

CLASSIFICATION

Sunscreen

ACTIONS

Protects skin from sunburn, photoaging, and photosensitivity reactions to certain drugs. Decreases the risk of actinic keratosis and skin cancer.

TYPES OF ULTRAVIOLET RADIATION

- UVA—penetrates both the epidermis and the dermis
  - Primary cause of immunosuppression, photosensitive drug reactions, photoaging of the skin (wrinkling, breakdown of elastic fibers)
  - Divided into UVA1 and UVA2
- UVB—penetrates only into the epidermis and is responsible for sunburn and tanning

TYPES OF SUNSCREENS

- **Organic (chemical) sunscreen**. Para-aminobenzoic acid (PABA), padimate O, cinnamates, salicylates, benzophenones, and avobenzone (Parsol 1789). Most of them absorb UVB and UVA2, but to absorb UVA1, the sunscreen must have avobenzone in the product.
- **Inorganic (physical) sunscreen**. Only two agents: titanium dioxide and zinc oxide. Act as a barrier to the sun's rays.

SUN PROTECTION FACTOR

- Sun protection factor (SPF) is an index of protection against UVB.
- Relationship between SPF and sunburn protection is not linear; that is, an SPF 30 does not indicate twice as much protection as an SPF 15.
- SPF 15 indicates a 93% block of UVB, SPF 30 indicates a 96.7% block, and SPF 40 indicates a 97.5% block.

SIDE EFFECTS

- Contact dermatitis and photosensitivity, especially with products containing PABA.
- PABA products should be avoided in patients allergic to benzocaine, sulfonamides, or thiazides.

NURSING IMPLICATIONS

1. Teach patient to use a sunscreen that covers both UVA and UVB (broad spectrum).
2. Teach patient to reapply sunscreen after swimming or profuse sweating.
3. Teach patient to avoid sun exposure in the middle of the day, especially between 10:00 a.m. and 4:00 p.m.
4. Encourage other protection measures, such as wearing a broad-brimmed hat, sunglasses, and protective clothing and finding shade when outside.
5. Explain SPF and encourage use of a sunscreen with SPF 30.

ANTIGOUT

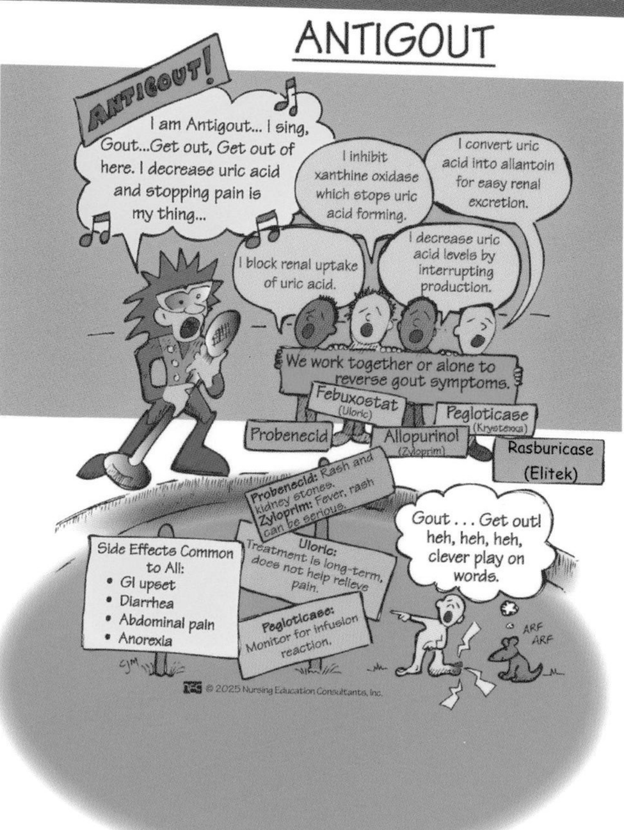
ANTIGOUT!
I am Antigout... I sing, Gout...Get out, Get out of here. I decrease uric acid and stopping pain is my thing...
I inhibit xanthine oxidase which stops uric acid forming.
I convert uric acid into allantoin for easy renal excretion.
I block renal uptake of uric acid.
I decrease uric acid levels by interrupting production.
We work together or alone to reverse gout symptoms.
Febuxostat (Uloric)
Pegloticase (Krystexxa)
Probenecid
Allopurinol (Zyloprim)
Rasburicase (Elitek)
Probenecid: Rash and kidney stones. Zyloprim: Fever, rash can be serious.
Side Effects Common to All:
• GI upset
• Diarrhea
• Abdominal pain
• Anorexia
Uloric: Treatment is long-term, does not help relieve pain.
Pegloticase: Monitor for infusion reaction.
Gout . . . Get out! heh, heh, heh, clever play on words.
ARF ARF
© 2025 Nursing Education Consultants, Inc.

What You Need to Know

Antigout Agents

EXAMPLES

Febuxostat (Uloric), allopurinol (Zyloprim), probenecid, pegloticase (Krystexxa), rasburicase (Elitek), colchicine (Colcrys)

ACTIONS

Note: Some medications are ■ **Black Box Warning** *and/or* ▲ **High Alert.**
Xanthine oxidase inhibitors (febuxostat, allopurinol) inhibit uric acid formation. Uricosuric agent (probenecid) accelerates uric acid excretion. Recombinant uric acid oxidase (pegloticase, rasburicase) promotes uric acid breakdown. Colchicine is used primarily for patients who do not respond to other safer agents.

USES

- Long-term treatment of acute gouty arthritis; not useful in the treatment of an acute attack of gouty arthritis
- Pegloticase—not used readily because of significant risks for adverse effects and high cost
- Rasburicase—treats hyperuricemia associated with cancer chemotherapy
- Nonsteroidal anti-inflammatory drugs (preferred) and prednisone—treat *acute* gout flares

CONTRAINDICATIONS AND PRECAUTIONS

- Severe gastrointestinal (GI) cardiac, hepatic, or kidney disorders
- Aspirin and other salicylates should not be given with probenecid

SIDE EFFECTS

- Febuxostat (Uloric): nausea, arthralgia, rash, and abnormal liver function studies
- Probenecid: vomiting, nausea, anorexia; renal deposits of urate may cause damage
- Allopurinol (Zyloprim): GI symptoms, drowsiness, headache, abdominal cramping; toxicity—hypersensitivity syndrome with rash, fever, eosinophilia, and liver and kidney malfunction; prolonged use may cause cataracts
- Pegloticase (Krystexxa): anaphylaxis, infusion reactions
- Rasburicase (Elitek): vomiting, fever, nausea, neutropenia
- Colchicine (Colcrys): GI upset, myelosuppression

NURSING IMPLICATIONS

1. Hyperuricemic (antigout) agents are given to prevent an attack; they are not effective for an acute attack.
2. Initially, symptoms may worsen until uric acid levels are decreased.
3. Antigout agents can be given with food and milk to decrease GI discomfort.
4. Advise patient to avoid grapefruit juice with colchicine.
5. Teach lifestyle changes—controlling weight, limiting alcohol consumption, limiting meals with meats and fish rich in purines, increasing low-fat dairy consumption, and consuming cherries.
6. Encourage an increased intake of fluids to increase excretion of uric acid and to decrease plasma concentration.

DISEASE-MODIFYING ANTIRHEUMATIC DRUGS (DMARDs)

To Reduce Joint Destruction and Slow Progression of Rheumatoid Arthritis

Nonbiologic

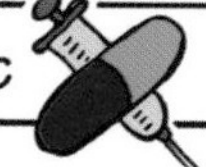

hyDroxychloroquine (Plaquenil)
Methotrexate, Minocycline (Minocin)
Arava (Leflunomide)
imuRan (Azathioprine)
golD salts
Sulfasalazine (Azulfidine)

Biologic

aDalimumab (Humira)
certolizuMab (Cimzia)
Abatacept (Orencia)
etaneRcept (Enbrel)
remicaDe (Infliximab)
Simponi (Golimumab)

Blood tests that need monitoring – CBC, LFT

Patient Education:

- Report immediately signs and symptoms of infection, bleeding, shortness of breath, or dysuria.
- Alcohol should be avoided while the patient is on methotrexate.
- The patient should avoid prolonged exposure to sunlight.
- Methotrexate must be stored at room temperature.

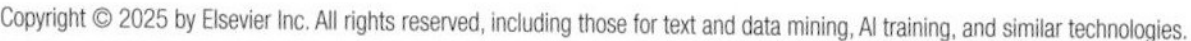

What You Need to Know

Disease-Modifying Antirheumatic Drugs (DMARDs)

TYPES

- **Nonbiologic (traditional) disease-modifying antirheumatic drugs (DMARDs)**: methotrexate (Rheumatrex, Trexall), sulfasalazine (Azulfidine), leflunomide (Arava), hydroxychloroquine (Plaquenil), minocycline (Minocin), penicillamine (Cuprimine), gold salts, azathioprine (Imuran), cyclosporine (Sandimmune), protein A column (Prosorba)
- **Biologic DMARDs**: *tumor necrosis factor (TNF) antagonists* (adalimumab [Humira], etanercept [Enbrel]); *B-lymphocyte-depleting agents* (rituximab [Rituxan]); *T-cell activation inhibitors* (abatacept [Orencia]); *interleukin-6 receptor antagonists* (tocilizumab [Actemra]); *interleukin-1 receptor antagonists* (anakinra [Kineret])

ACTIONS

Note: Some medications are ■ **Black Box Warning** *and/or* ▲ **High Alert.**

Reduce joint destruction and slow disease progression of rheumatoid arthritis.

USES

- Treats rheumatoid arthritis (usually started within 3 months of diagnosis)
- Methotrexate is the first-line therapy

SIDE EFFECTS

- TNF antagonists and other biologic DMARDs—serious infections (bacterial sepsis, invasive fungal infections, tuberculosis, hepatitis B virus infection), cancer, hematologic disorders, severe allergic reactions, injection site reactions (pain, redness, swelling)
- Methotrexate—hepatic fibrosis, bone marrow suppression, GI ulceration, pneumonitis
- Hydroxychloroquine—retinal damage (often irreversible leading to blindness)

NURSING IMPLICATIONS

1. Teach patient about signs of infection and to report promptly.
2. Monitor for side effects.
3. Administer folic acid with methotrexate as prescribed to minimize GI and hepatic toxicity.
4. Monitor (complete blood count, platelet count, liver and kidney function).
5. Advise patient to avoid live virus vaccines.
6. Teach patient and family how to administer a subcutaneous injection with etanercept and other TNF antagonists.

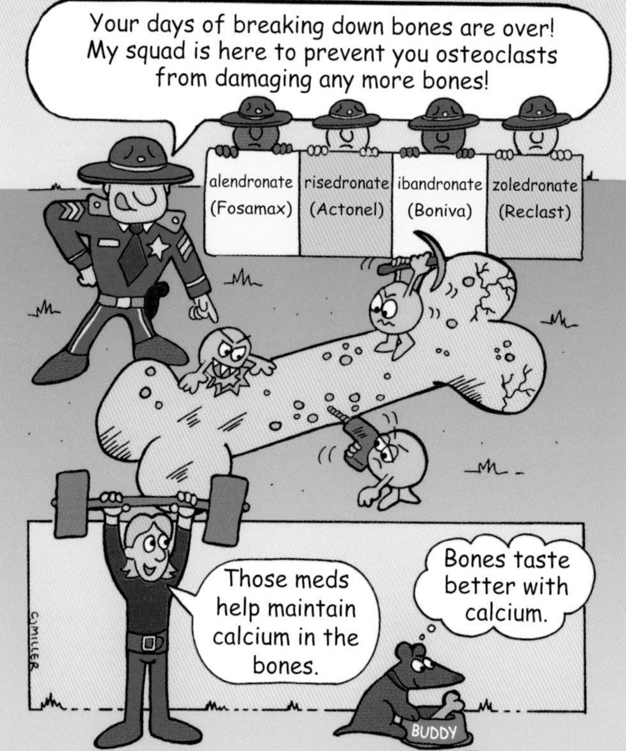
BISPHOSPHONATE THERAPY
Your days of breaking down bones are over! My squad is here to prevent you osteoclasts from damaging any more bones!
alendronate (Fosamax)
risedronate (Actonel)
ibandronate (Boniva)
zoledronate (Reclast)
Those meds help maintain calcium in the bones.
Bones taste better with calcium.
BUDDY
C.J. MILLER
© 2025 Nursing Education Consultants, Inc.

What You Need to Know

Bisphosphonate Therapy

EXAMPLES

Alendronate (Fosamax), risedronate (Actonel), ibandronate (Boniva), zoledronate (Reclast). (*Note: The "dronate" ending for the bisphosphonates.*)

CLASSIFICATION

Bisphosphonate, bone resorption inhibitor

ACTIONS

Incorporated into the bone and inhibits bone resorption by decreasing activity of osteoclasts; provides significant increase in bone mineral density

USES

- Prevents and treats the progression of osteoporosis in postmenopausal women
- Treats Paget disease in men and women
- Treats osteoporosis in men
- Treats glucocorticoid-induced osteoporosis in men and women
- Treats hypercalcemia of malignancy

CONTRAINDICATIONS AND PRECAUTIONS

- GI irritation, esophageal disease, gastroesophageal reflux disease, and renal function impairment
- Patients with swallowing disorders

SIDE EFFECTS

- Oral medications—esophagitis, GI irritation and discomfort, back pain
- Atypical fractures (femoral), ocular inflammation, musculoskeletal pain, osteonecrosis of the jaw (rare)
- Fever with flu-like symptoms—zoledronate

NURSING IMPLICATIONS

1. Oral medications—patient should take each tablet or oral solution in the morning with a full glass of water (6–8 oz) at least 30 to 60 minutes before the first bite of food, beverage, or medication of the day. Orange juice, coffee, or food significantly decreases effectiveness.
2. Teach patient not chew or suck on the tablet.
3. After taking medication, the patient should remain upright (sitting or standing) for 30 to 60 minutes. Teach patient to not lie down until after eating.
4. Teach patient to not take medication at bedtime or at the same time as other medications (including aspirin, antacids, or calcium supplements).
5. Teach patient to wait at least 30 minutes before taking any other drug.
6. Boniva is taken once a month; however, the previous precautions are still necessary on administration.

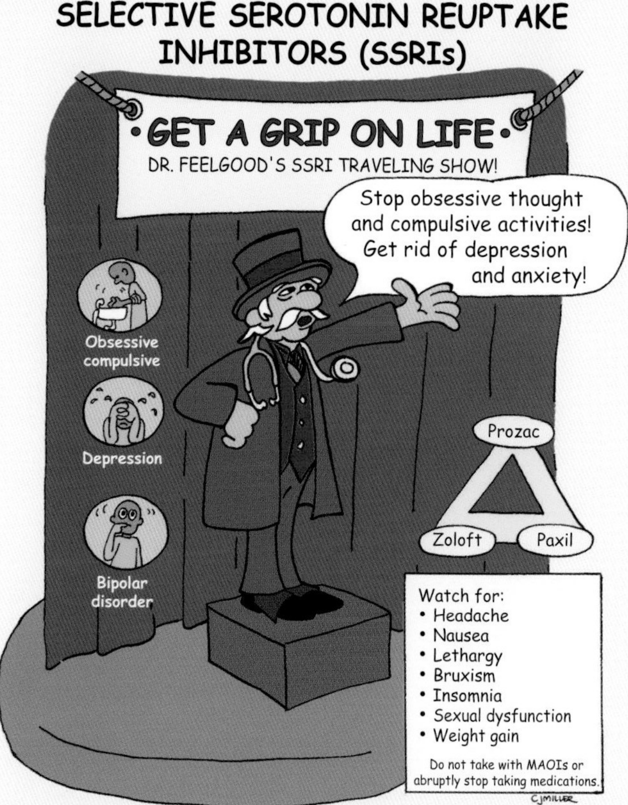
SELECTIVE SEROTONIN REUPTAKE INHIBITORS (SSRIs)
•GET A GRIP ON LIFE•
DR. FEELGOOD'S SSRI TRAVELING SHOW!
Stop obsessive thought and compulsive activities! Get rid of depression and anxiety!
Obsessive compulsive
Depression
Bipolar disorder
Prozac
Zoloft
Paxil
Watch for:
• Headache
• Nausea
• Lethargy
• Bruxism
• Insomnia
• Sexual dysfunction
• Weight gain
Do not take with MAOIs or abruptly stop taking medications.
CJMILLER

What You Need to Know

Selective Serotonin Reuptake Inhibitors

EXAMPLES

Fluoxetine (Prozac), paroxetine (Paxil), sertraline (Zoloft), fluvoxamine (Luvox), escitalopram (Lexapro), and citalopram (Celexa)

ACTIONS ■ Black Box Warning

Selective serotonin reuptake inhibitors (SSRIs) decrease the reuptake of serotonin at selected nerve terminals in the central nervous system (CNS) and increase serotonin activity at the nerve synapse. Increased availability of serotonin at the receptors results in mood elevation and reduced anxiety.

USES

- Major depression, bipolar disorder, obsessive-compulsive disorder, panic disorder, bulimia nervosa, and premenstrual dysphoric disorder

CONTRAINDICATIONS AND PRECAUTIONS

- Hypersensitivity to SSRIs
- Concurrent use of monoamine oxidase inhibitors (MAOIs)

SIDE EFFECTS

- Nausea, insomnia, weight gain, nervousness, anxiety, headache
- Sexual dysfunction: decreased libido, impotence, delayed ejaculation, delayed or absent orgasm
- Hyponatremia (primarily in older adults), neonatal abstinence syndrome and persistent pulmonary hypertension of the newborn, increased risk of gastrointestinal (GI) bleeding, bruxism (clenching and grinding of teeth)
- Serotonin syndrome: agitation, confusion, disorientation, hallucinations; deaths have occurred

NURSING IMPLICATIONS

1. Treatment of depression places the patient at increased risk for suicide; monitor the patient for mood and behavioral changes.
2. Do not stop taking medication; withdrawal should be gradual, not abrupt.
3. Patient should advise health care provider (HCP) if she might be pregnant; SSRIs are not recommended for use during pregnancy or lactation.
4. Bleeding problems may occur if used concurrently with anticoagulants, antiplatelets, or nonsteroidal anti-inflammatory drugs (NSAIDs).
5. Teach patient that it may take 4 weeks or longer for the full effect of the medication to occur.
6. Teach patient and family about the side effects and advise them to notify the HCP if any symptoms occur.

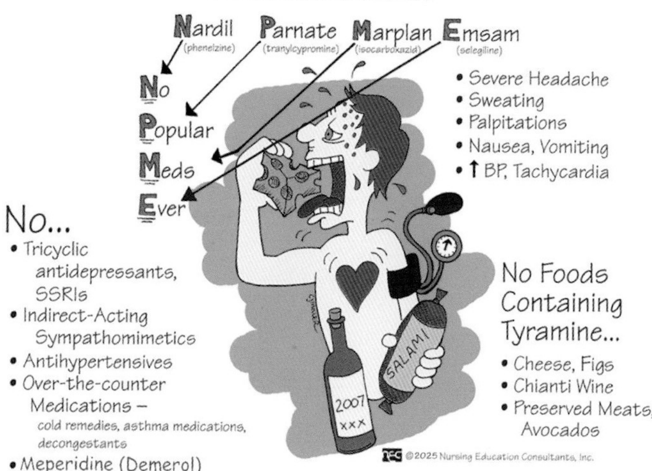
MAO INHIBITORS
Nardil
(phenelzine)
Parnate
(tranylcypromine)
Marplan
(isocarboxazid)
Emsam
(selegiline)
No
Popular
Meds
Ever
• Severe Headache
• Sweating
• Palpitations
• Nausea, Vomiting
• ↑ BP, Tachycardia
No...
• Tricyclic antidepressants, SSRIs
• Indirect-Acting Sympathomimetics
• Antihypertensives
• Over-the-counter Medications –
cold remedies, asthma medications, decongestants
• Meperidine (Demerol)
No Foods Containing Tyramine...
• Cheese, Figs
• Chianti Wine
• Preserved Meats, Avocados
SALAMI
2007
XXX
©2025 Nursing Education Consultants, Inc.

What You Need to Know

Monoamine Oxidase Inhibitors

EXAMPLES

Phenelzine (Nardil), tranylcypromine (Parnate), isocarboxazid (Marplan), selegiline (Emsam)

ACTION

The antidepressant effects of the MAOIs are the result of blocking monoamine oxidase in nerve terminals. This action increases the availability and concentration of norepinephrine (NE) and serotonin for neurotransmission.

USES

- MAOIs are reserved for patients with atypical depression and who have not responded to tricyclic antidepressants (TCAs) and SSRIs.

CONTRAINDICATIONS AND PRECAUTIONS

- Impaired kidney or hepatic function.
- Cardiovascular and/or cerebrovascular disease.
- Concurrent use with SSRIs or TCAs.
- Hypertensive crisis can be triggered by eating foods rich in tyramine and medications containing diuretics, antihistamines, antihypertensives, ephedrine.
- MAOIs interact with many medications.

SIDE EFFECTS

- CNS stimulation: anxiety, agitation, hypomania, mania
- Skin rash may occur with application of transdermal selegiline
- Orthostatic hypotension
- Hypertensive crisis from dietary tyramine: headache, tachycardia, palpitations, nausea, vomiting, sweating

NURSING IMPLICATIONS

1. Advise patient to avoid all prescription and over-the-counter drugs that have not been approved by the health care professional, especially cold remedies, nasal decongestants, and asthma medications.
2. Advise patients to tell all health care professionals they are taking an MAOI.
3. Assess patient for changes in mood and suicidal ideation.
4. Advise patient to change positions slowly to minimize hypotension.
5. Teach patient to avoid tyramine-rich foods that can lead to hypertensive crisis (fermented meats [smoked sausage, pepperoni, salami, bologna], dried or cured fish, all cheeses, Chianti wine, some imported beers, foods with yeast extract, dietary supplements with protein extract, soy sauce, ripe avocados, figs, bananas) and ginseng, chocolate, caffeine.

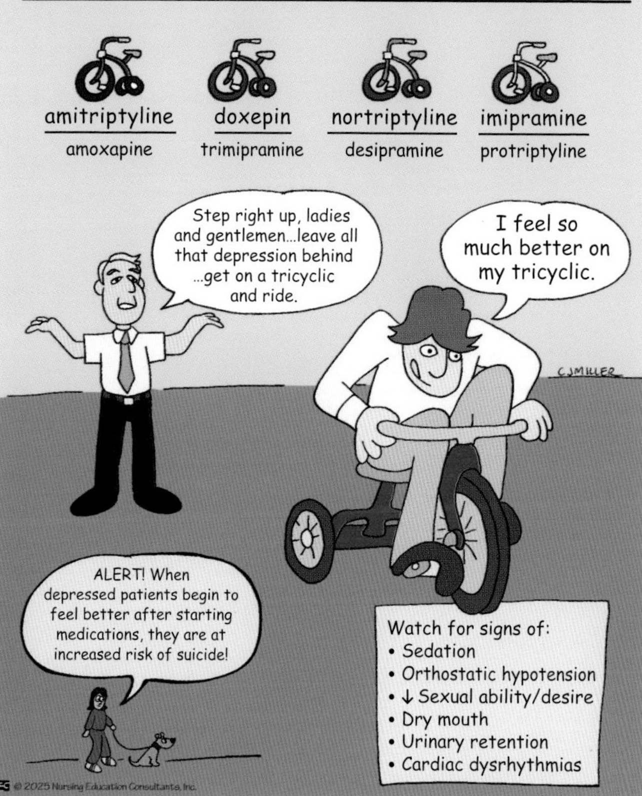
TRICYCLIC ANTIDEPRESSANTS (TCAs)
amitriptyline
amoxapine
doxepin
trimipramine
nortriptyline
desipramine
imipramine
protriptyline
Step right up, ladies and gentlemen...leave all that depression behind ...get on a tricyclic and ride.
I feel so much better on my tricyclic.
CJMILLER
ALERT! When depressed patients begin to feel better after starting medications, they are at increased risk of suicide!
Watch for signs of:
• Sedation
• Orthostatic hypotension
• ↓ Sexual ability/desire
• Dry mouth
• Urinary retention
• Cardiac dysrhythmias
© 2025 Nursing Education Consultants, Inc.

What You Need to Know

Tricyclic Antidepressants (TCAs)

ACTION ■ Black Box Warning

Amitriptyline, doxepin, imipramine, and trimipramine block reabsorption of NE and serotonin, which allows more of the neurotransmitters to be available at postsynaptic receptors. Desipramine, nortriptyline, protriptyline, and amoxapine only block reuptake of NE; amoxapine also blocks receptors for dopamine.

USES

- Not used as often as in the past; considered a second-line drug
- Depression, bipolar disorder, fibromyalgia syndrome
- Neuropathic pain, chronic insomnia, attention-deficit/hyperactivity disorder (ADHD), panic disorder, obsessive-compulsive disorder

CONTRAINDICATIONS

- History of coronary heart disease, heart failure, dysrhythmias
- Not administered within 14 days of taking MAOI
- Glaucoma or urinary retention (doxepin)

PRECAUTIONS

- History of suicidal behavior, seizures, hyperthyroidism, diabetes
- Cardiac, kidney, hepatic disease; urinary retention

SIDE EFFECTS

- Sedation, orthostatic hypotension, diaphoresis, anticholinergic effects (dry mouth, urinary retention, blurred vision)
- Cardiotoxicity: decreases vagal influence and slows conduction (dysrhythmias)

NURSING IMPLICATIONS

1. Teach patient how to manage orthostatic hypotension; notify HCP for persistent low blood pressure (BP) or rapid pulse rate.
2. Administer at bedtime to minimize problems with sedation.
3. Advise patient to stop smoking and to avoid CNS depressants (alcohol, antihistamines, opioids, sedatives).
4. Antidepressant effects will not peak for several weeks and therapy usually continues for a minimum of 6 months; do not abruptly stop taking medication or a relapse may occur.
5. When a depressed patient begins to feel better, the risk of suicide increases; monitor patient closely for mood changes or unusual changes in behavior.

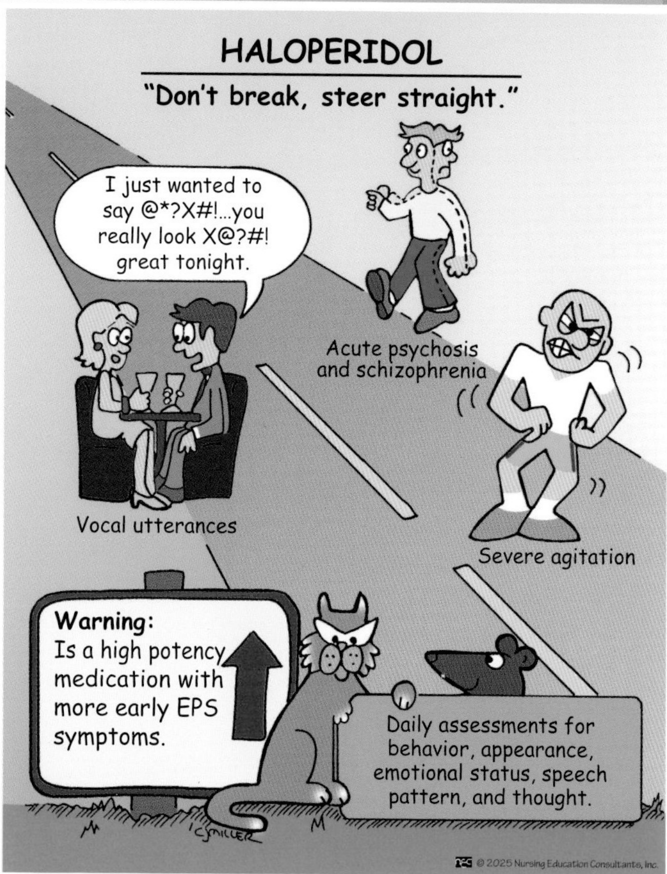
HALOPERIDOL
"Don't break, steer straight."
I just wanted to say @*?X#!...you really look X@?#! great tonight.
Acute psychosis and schizophrenia
Vocal utterances
Severe agitation
Warning: Is a high potency medication with more early EPS symptoms.
Daily assessments for behavior, appearance, emotional status, speech pattern, and thought.
© 2025 Nursing Education Consultants, Inc.

What You Need to Know

Haloperidol

ACTION ■ Black Box Warning

A first-generation antipsychotic that blocks receptors for DA within the CNS as well as outside the CNS.

USES

- Schizophrenia, acute psychosis, Tourette disorder
- Emergency sedation of patients who are severely agitated

CONTRAINDICATIONS AND PRECAUTIONS

- Parkinson disease (will counteract effectiveness of Parkinson medications and increase the symptoms), bone marrow depression, coma, older adults with dementia-related psychosis
- History of seizures, dysrhythmias, myocardial infarction, or heart failure
- Glaucoma, kidney and hepatic dysfunction, prostatic hypertrophy
- Electrolyte imbalances (hypokalemia and hypomagnesemia)

SIDE EFFECTS

- Extrapyramidal symptoms (EPS)

Early symptoms:

- Parkinsonism (bradykinesia, masklike facies, drooling, tremor, gait problems)
- Acute dystonia (spasms of tongue, face, neck, back)
- Akathisia (compulsive restless movement, anxiety, agitation)

Late symptoms:

- Tardive dyskinesia (twisting movement of face and tongue; "lip smacking"; involuntary movement of extremities and trunk); symptoms often irreversible
- Neuroleptic malignant syndrome (rare but serious)
  - "Lead pipe" rigidity, high fever, sweating, dysrhythmias, BP fluctuations, death
- Anticholinergic effects: drowsiness, dry mouth, constipation, urinary retention
- Prolonged QT interval and potential for dysrhythmias

NURSING IMPLICATIONS

1. Frequently monitor patient for reduction of target symptoms.
2. Routinely assess for presence of involuntary movement associated with early and late symptoms of EPS.
3. Teach patient to avoid skin contact with the oral liquid preparations because they may cause contact dermatitis.
4. Patient should avoid sunlight, apply sunscreen, and wear protective clothing.

ALZHEIMER'S DISEASE (AD) DRUGS

When It's Difficult to Stay in Touch

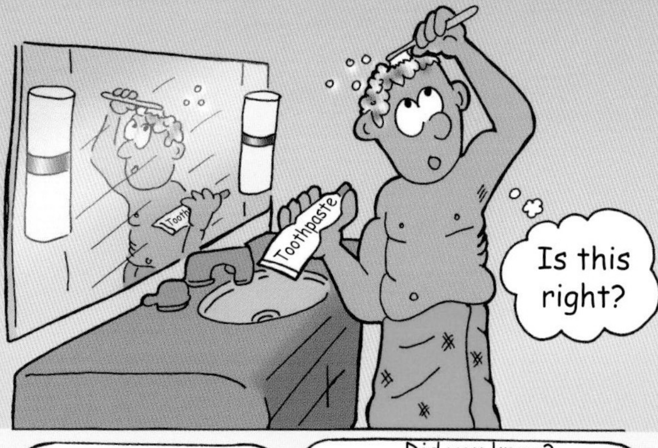

These drugs do not stop the progression of Alzheimer's disease but may improve cognitive function.

Did you know? After age 65 years, the risk of AD doubles every 10 years until age 85 to 90 years, then levels off or declines.

CJMILLER

What You Need to Know

Alzheimer Disease Drugs (AD)

CLASSIFICATION

Cholinesterase inhibitors for mild-to-moderate AD are donepezil (Aricept), rivastigmine (Exelon), and galantamine (Razadyne). Memantine (Namenda) is the only *N-methyl-D-aspartate (NMDA) receptor antagonists* for moderate-to-severe AD.

ACTIONS ■ Black Box Warning

Cholinesterase inhibitors: inhibit breakdown of acetylcholine (ACh) by acetylcholinesterase. This breakdown increases the availability of ACh for improved nerve transmission by the central cholinergic neurons.
NMDA receptor antagonists: decreases effects of glutamate (principal excitatory neurotransmitter) at NMDA receptors in the brain. Persistent CNS excitation by glutamate is associated with symptoms of AD.

USES

- Slows progression of AD symptoms; does not stop progression or cure underlying disease process; donepezil and memantine are the only drugs approved for severe symptoms.

PRECAUTIONS

- Patients with asthma or chronic obstructive pulmonary disease may experience bronchoconstriction caused by increased levels of ACh.
- Urine alkalinizing agents (i.e., sodium bicarbonate, potassium citrate) can increase risk of toxicity with memantine.

SIDE EFFECTS

- Cholinergic effects
  - GI: nausea, vomiting, dyspepsia, diarrhea
  - Bronchoconstriction, dizziness, headache, confusion (memantine)
  - Bradycardia—leading to fainting, increased patient falls, fall-related fractures
- Toxic effects: cholinergic crisis; atropine is antidote for cholinergic crisis

NURSING IMPLICATIONS

1. Obtain baseline assessment of cognitive function to determine response to medication.
2. Assess for urinary obstruction and monitor for difficulty urinating.
3. Monitor for respiratory airway compromise and bradycardia.
4. May be taken with or without food; administer donepezil at bedtime
5. Do not crush or chew memantine; swallow whole or place contents of drug in soft food like applesauce.
6. Explain to family that these drugs are not a cure, but only slow the progression of symptoms.

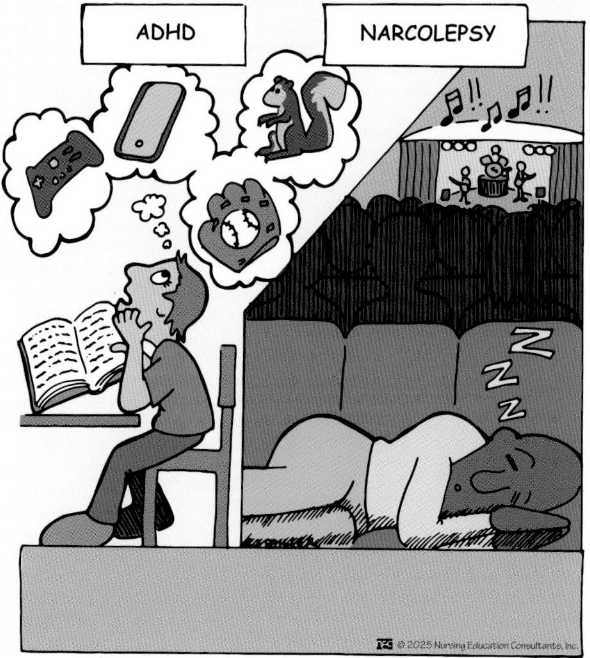
CNS STIMULANTS
SYMPTOM MANAGEMENT OF
ADHD
NARCOLEPSY
© 2025 Nursing Education Consultants, Inc.

What You Need to Know

CNS Stimulants

EXAMPLES

ADHD—methylphenidate (Ritalin), dextroamphetamine/amphetamine (Adderall), dexmethylphenidate (Focalin), lisdexamfetamine (Vyvanse)
Narcolepsy—methylphenidate (Ritalin), modafinil (Provigil), armodafinil (Nuvigil), solriamfetol (Sunosi), pitolisant (Wakix)

ACTION

Promote the neuronal release of norepinephrine (NE) and dopamine (DA) and partly blocking NE and DA reuptake in the CNS and peripheral nerves.

USES

- Attention—deficit/hyperactivity disorder (ADHD)
- Narcolepsy—disorder characterized by excessive daytime sleepiness and falling asleep suddenly

CONTRAINDICATIONS AND PRECAUTIONS

- Hypertension, hyperthyroidism, agitated states
- Cardiovascular disease, advanced atherosclerosis
- History of drug abuse and being on an MAOI

SIDE EFFECTS

- Insomnia, restlessness, weight loss, growth suppression in children
- Palpitations, hypertension, angina, dysrhythmias
- Tolerance and physical dependence develop with regular use
- Withdrawal reaction—extreme fatigue, depression
- Hypersensitivity reaction—erythema, edema, papules, vesicles

NURSING IMPLICATIONS

1. Teach patient to swallow long-acting medications without crushing or chewing.
2. Teach patient using transdermal preparations to apply one patch to alternating hips each morning and to remove each patch not more than 9 hours after applying.
3. Monitor children with ADHD for a reduction in symptoms (impulsiveness, hyperactivity, and inattention) and improvement in cognitive function.
4. Monitor for a reduction in daytime sleepiness in patients with narcolepsy.
5. In children, administer medication during or after meals to improve growth reduction by minimizing appetite suppression.
6. "Drug holidays," which is not taking the medication on weekends and during the summer are recommended by some HCPs.

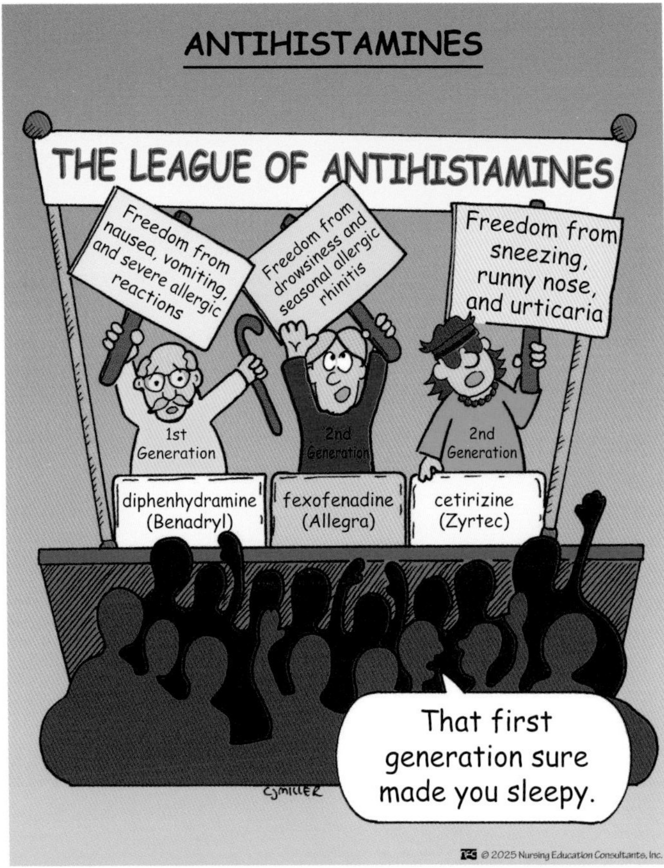

ANTIHISTAMINES

THE LEAGUE OF ANTIHISTAMINES

Freedom from nausea, vomiting, and severe allergic reactions

Freedom from drowsiness and seasonal allergic rhinitis

Freedom from sneezing, runny nose, and urticaria

1st Generation

2nd Generation

2nd Generation

diphenhydramine (Benadryl)

fexofenadine (Allegra)

cetirizine (Zyrtec)

That first generation sure made you sleepy.

CJMILLER

What You Need to Know

Antihistamines

ACTIONS

Competitively block the H_1-receptor sites and impede histamine-mediated responses. Second-generation antihistamines cause less drowsiness.

USES

- Prevent and treat seasonal allergies; decrease itching (pruritus)
- Are adjuncts used with epinephrine for severe allergic reactions (anaphylaxis)
- Prevent and treat motion sickness and insomnia

CONTRAINDICATIONS AND PRECAUTIONS

- Asthma—acute or chronic; chronic obstructive pulmonary disease (COPD)
- Pregnancy and lactation; hypertension
- Conditions resulting in urinary retention and obstruction

SIDE EFFECTS

- *First generation:* frequently cause sedation and anticholinergic effects
  - *Diphenhydramine (Benadryl):* side effects include sedation, thickening of bronchial secretions, dry mouth, drowsiness, dizziness, muscular weakness; may cause paradoxical reaction in children—restlessness, anxiety
  - Other example: *chlorpheniramine (Chlor-Trimeton)*
- *Second generation:* Minimal side effects occur—drowsiness, dry mouth, constipation, urinary retention, headache
  - *Cetirizine (Zyrtec):* may cause paradoxical reaction in children—restlessness, anxiety; more sedative effect than other second-generation drugs
  - *Fexofenadine (Allegra):* certain fruit juices (apple, orange, grapefruit) can reduce the absorption of the medication
  - *Loratadine (Claritin):* may cause photosensitivity reactions (avoid direct exposure to sunlight)

NURSING IMPLICATIONS

1. Caution patient not to take antihistamines with alcohol and other central nervous system (CNS) depressants.
2. Caution patient about drowsiness because of safety concerns.
3. Do not administer antihistamines within 4 days of skin testing.
4. Teach patient to take with food if gastrointestinal (GI) upset occurs.
5. Advise patient to exercise extreme caution when driving or performing other hazardous activities.
6. Using sugar-free hard candy or taking frequent sips of water can reduce dry mouth.
7. Teach patient to avoid certain fruit juices in the interval between 4 hours before dosing and 1 to 2 hours after dosing if taking Allegra.

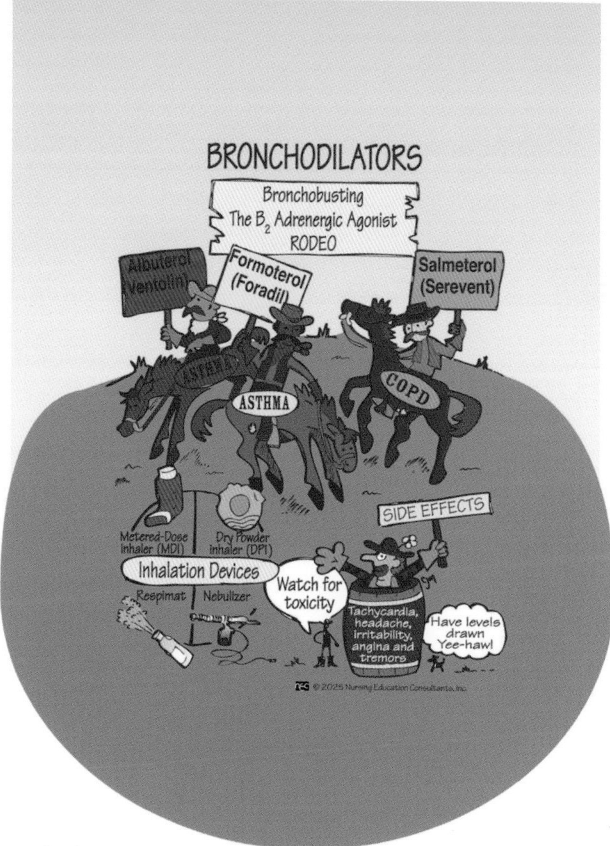

BRONCHODILATORS
Bronchobusting
The B_2 Adrenergic Agonist
RODEO
Albuterol (Ventolin)
Formoterol (Foradil)
Salmeterol (Serevent)
ASTHMA
ASTHMA
COPD
Metered-Dose Inhaler (MDI)
Dry Powder Inhaler (DPI)
Inhalation Devices
Respimat
Nebulizer
SIDE EFFECTS
Watch for toxicity
Tachycardia, headache, irritability, angina and tremors
Have levels drawn Yee-haw!
© 2025 Nursing Education Consultants, Inc.

What You Need to Know

Bronchodilators

ACTIONS

Note: Some medications are ■ **Black Box Warning** and/or ▲ **High Alert.**

Beta$_2$-adrenergic agonists are sympathomimetic agents that relax the smooth muscles in the bronchioles, producing dilation and relieving bronchospasm.

TYPES

- Inhaled short-acting beta$_2$-agonists (SABAs): albuterol, levalbuterol
- Inhaled long-acting beta$_2$-agonists (LABAs): salmeterol, formoterol, arformoterol, indacaterol
- Oral agents: albuterol, terbutaline
  (*Note: The SABAs and LABAs have the suffix, "terol."*)

USES

- SABAs: treat acute exacerbations of asthma; prevent exercise-induced bronchospasm
- LABAs: preferred for patients with COPD; in patients with asthma, they are not first-line therapy and must be combined with a glucocorticoid
- Oral agents: long-term control for asthma; not first-line therapy

SIDE EFFECTS

- Headache, nausea, restlessness, nervousness, tremors
- Increased blood pressure, heartburn, insomnia, bronchial irritation

ADVERSE OR TOXIC EFFECTS (EXCESSIVE SYMPATHOMIMETIC STIMULATION)

- Palpitations, tachycardia, chest pain, seizures, tremor (oral preparations)

NURSING IMPLICATIONS

1. Evaluate patient's respiratory status and vital signs.
2. Explain to patient which type of medication is for long-term control and which one is for short-term response. SABAs are used to treat and/or to prevent immediate problems; LABAs are given on a schedule for maintenance.
3. LABA preparations are not recommended for aborting an ongoing asthmatic attack but are used when asthma is severe and are combined with a glucocorticoid, preferably in the same inhalation device.
4. Advise patient not to use more doses than ordered—can develop angina, tachydysrhythmias, seizures.
5. Check with health care provider before using over-the-counter (OTC) medicine.
6. Teach patient the correct use of inhalation devices—metered-dose inhaler (MDI), dry powder inhaler (DPI), Respimat (handheld inhaler delivers a fine mist of medication without the use of a propellant), nebulizer.

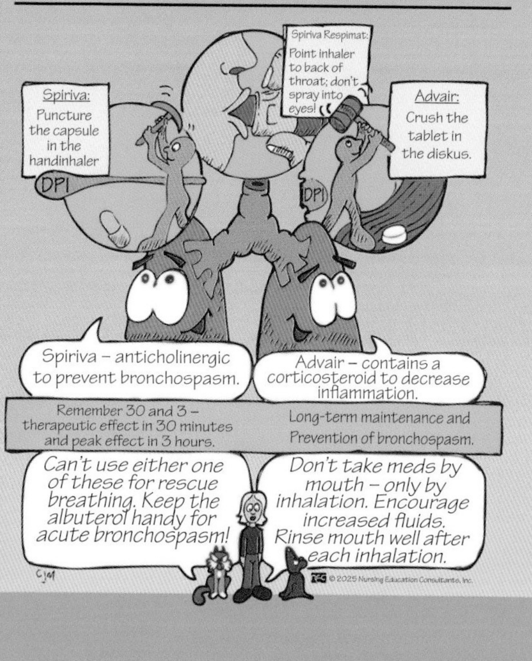
FLUTICASONE/SALMETEROL
TIOTROPIUM
Spiriva Respimat:
Point inhaler to back of throat; don't spray into eyes!
Spiriva:
Puncture the capsule in the handinhaler
Advair:
Crush the tablet in the diskus.
DPI
DPI
Spiriva – anticholinergic to prevent bronchospasm.
Advair – contains a corticosteroid to decrease inflammation.
Remember 30 and 3 – therapeutic effect in 30 minutes and peak effect in 3 hours.
Long-term maintenance and Prevention of bronchospasm.
Can't use either one of these for rescue breathing. Keep the albuterol handy for acute bronchospasm!
Don't take meds by mouth – only by inhalation. Encourage increased fluids. Rinse mouth well after each inhalation.
© 2025 Nursing Education Consultants, Inc.

What You Need to Know

Advair and Spiriva

FLUTICASONE/SALMETEROL (ADVAIR)

Classification
Glucocorticoid and LABA combination

ACTIONS ■ Black Box Warning

Provides anti-inflammatory and bronchodilator actions

DOSE

Administered by Advair Diskus DPI one inhalation twice daily or as Advair HFA with an MDI, two inhalations twice daily.

TIOTROPIUM (SPIRIVA)

Classification
Anticholinergic bronchodilator

ACTIONS

Blocks muscarinic (cholinergic) receptors in the lung. Therapeutic effects begin in approximately 30 minutes, peak in 3 hours, and persist about 24 hours.

DOSE

Administered by Spiriva HandiHaler DPI in two inhalations (to ensure drug delivery of the entire contents of the capsule) once daily

USES

- Long-term control and maintenance treatment for prevention of bronchospasm and airway inflammation associated with asthma and COPD

SIDE EFFECTS

- Throat irritation, hoarseness, dry mouth, headache, angioedema
- Glucocorticoids—increased incidence of oropharyngeal fungal infections

NURSING IMPLICATIONS

1. Medications are to be taken every day as directed, even on days when patients feel they are breathing better.
2. Medications are not used for rescue in acute episodes.
3. Patients should carry a rescue inhaler, such as albuterol.
4. Advise patient to rinse mouth without swallowing after medication delivery of inhaled glucocorticoids to decrease risk of getting an oropharyngeal fungal infection (Advair).
5. Full effects of Spiriva make take a week or longer to be felt; however, lung function improvements may occur after the first dose.
6. Teach patient how to use the inhaler device.

ANTITUSSIVES, EXPECTORANTS, AND MUCOLYTICS

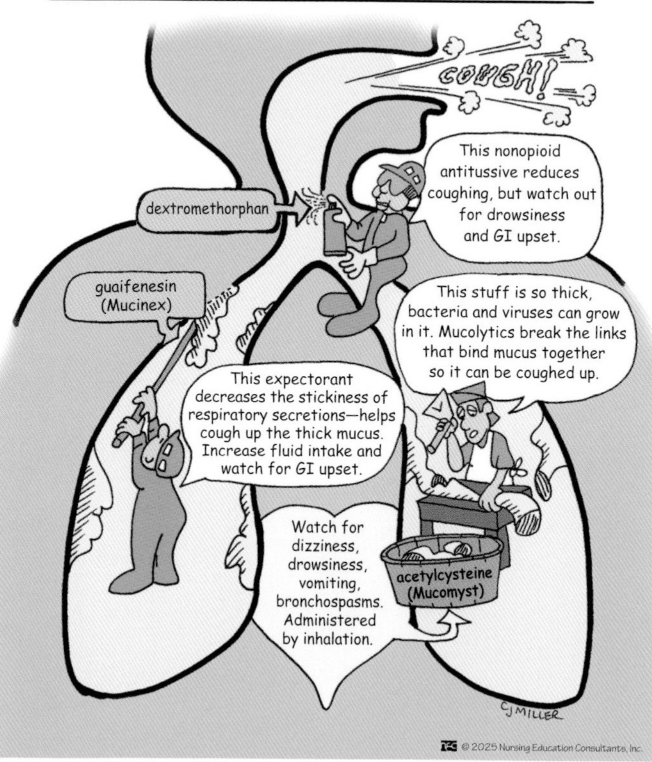

What You Need to Know

Antitussives, Expectorants, and Mucolytics

ACTION

Antitussives act either centrally (CNS) or locally in the peripheral nervous system to decrease irritation and suppress the cough response. *Expectorants* decrease the thickness of sputum and increase the ease of its removal for a productive cough. *Mucolytics* react directly with respiratory secretions by breaking up the mucus in the airways, making it easier to cough up.

USES

- *Antitussives* suppress cough
- *Expectorants* thin mucus and decrease viscosity (stickiness of mucus) to promote a more productive cough
- *Mucolytics* loosen and break down mucus making it easier to cough up

PRECAUTIONS

- Dextromethorphan is used in many OTC cough preparations.
- Origin of chronic cough should be investigated.
- Codeine is a very effective antitussive; is considered a Schedule V drug in cough medications and can suppress respiration.
- Codeine is not recommended for children under 12 years of age or for all pediatric patients undergoing tonsillectomy and/or adenoidectomy.
- Avoid OTC cough and cold remedies in children younger than 4–6 years of age.

SIDE EFFECTS

- *Antitussives:* dextromethorphan—euphoria (may be abused); codeine—drowsiness, constipation, GI upset, respiratory depression
- *Expectorants:* guaifenesin—nausea and vomiting, GI upset
- *Mucolytics:* acetylcysteine—nausea, rhinorrhea, dizziness, may trigger bronchospasms

NURSING IMPLICATIONS

1. Evaluate patient's respiratory status and response to medication.
2. Warn patient to avoid driving and operating machinery when taking codeine cough suppressant.
3. Encourage patient to increase intake of fluids; helps thin and loosen mucus.
4. Mucomyst has a short-term disagreeable odor (rotten eggs).
5. Teach patient to read labels; cold remedies are frequently combined with other drugs and may contain two or more of the following: nasal decongestant, antitussive, analgesic, antihistamine, and caffeine.

DRUGS FOR CERVICAL RIPENING: PROSTAGLANDINS

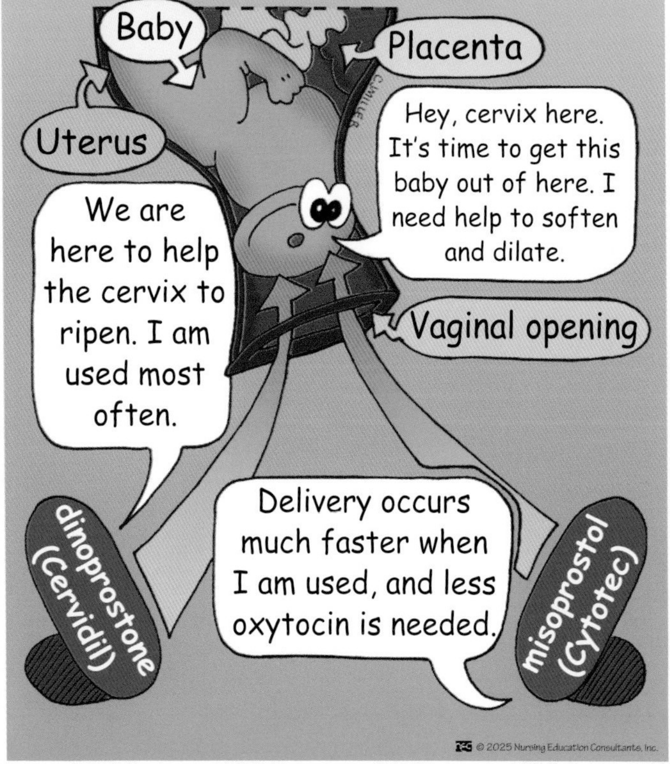

Baby

Placenta

Uterus

Hey, cervix here. It's time to get this baby out of here. I need help to soften and dilate.

We are here to help the cervix to ripen. I am used most often.

Vaginal opening

dinoprostone (Cervidil)

Delivery occurs much faster when I am used, and less oxytocin is needed.

misoprostol (Cytotec)

What You Need to Know

Drugs for Cervical Ripening: Prostaglandins

CLASSIFICATION

Prostaglandin

ACTIONS ■ Black Box Warning

Promote cervical ripening and act on the uterus to promote contractions

USES

- Preinduction cervical ripening when Bishop score is 4 or less
- Induction of labor when pregnancy has continued beyond 42 weeks
- Early induction of labor from complication(s)—abruptio placentae, premature rupture of the membranes, preeclampsia, eclampsia, gestational diabetes, fetal compromise or fetal demise

CONTRAINDICATIONS

- Umbilical cord prolapse, previous cesarean delivery
- Transverse fetal position, active genital herpes infection
- Placenta previa, history of removal of uterine fibroids

TYPES OF PREPARATIONS

- Dinoprostone
  - Gel (Prepidil): prefilled syringe administered intracervically by health care provider (HCP) using an endocervical catheter; may need more than one dose
  - Vaginal insert (Cervidil): vaginal pouch with a long tape containing drug is inserted vaginally; tape permits rapid removal of pouch if needed; only one dose given (pouch inserted) and is removed after 12 hours
  - Follow manufacturer guidelines for proper storage and handling of drug
- Misoprostol (Cytotec)
  - Tablet is inserted vaginally

SIDE EFFECTS

- Nausea, vomiting, diarrhea, fever
- Tachysystole: more than five contractions in 10 minutes (averaged over a 30-minute window)

NURSING IMPLICATIONS

1. Continuously monitor uterine activity (frequency, duration, strength of contractions) and fetal heart rate.
2. Oxytocin may be given 6 to 12 hours after last dinoprostone (Prepidil) gel dose or 30 minutes after Cervidil vaginal insert (pouch).
3. Teach patient that she should remain supine for at least 2 hours after Cervidil pouch is inserted.

OXYTOCIN (PITOCIN)

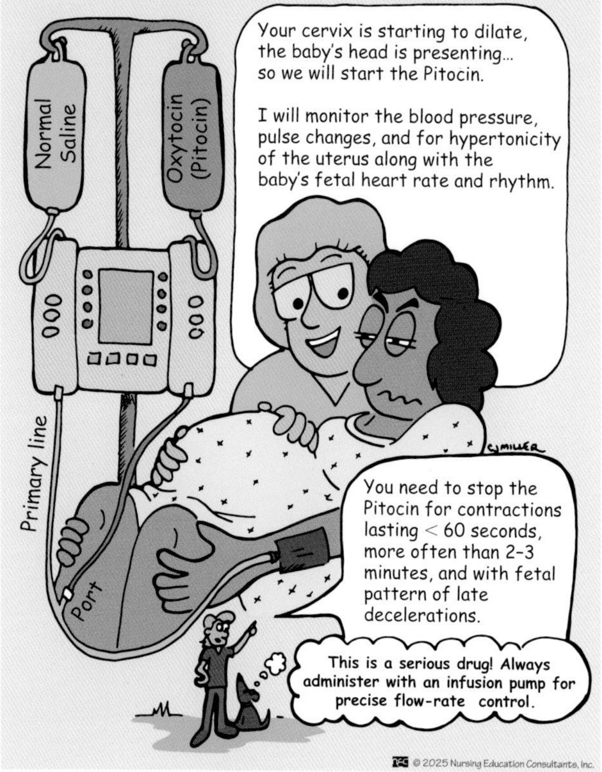

Normal Saline

Oxytocin (Pitocin)

Your cervix is starting to dilate, the baby's head is presenting... so we will start the Pitocin.

I will monitor the blood pressure, pulse changes, and for hypertonicity of the uterus along with the baby's fetal heart rate and rhythm.

Primary line

Port

CJMILLER

You need to stop the Pitocin for contractions lasting < 60 seconds, more often than 2-3 minutes, and with fetal pattern of late decelerations.

This is a serious drug! Always administer with an infusion pump for precise flow-rate control.

What You Need to Know

Oxytocin (Pitocin)

CLASSIFICATION

Hormone

ACTIONS ■ Black Box Warning ▲ High Alert

Contracts uterine muscle and stimulates the milk ejection reflex. Increases force, frequency, and duration of uterine contractions.

USES

- Inducing term labor
- Controlling postpartum hemorrhage
- Managing incomplete or inevitable abortion

CONTRAINDICATIONS

- Cephalopelvic disproportion, previous uterine surgery
- Unengaged fetal head, unfavorable fetal position or presentation
- Fetal distress without evidence of imminent delivery
- Placenta previa, umbilical cord prolapse
- Women with active genital herpes

PRECAUTIONS

- Used with great caution in women with high parity (five or more pregnancies)

SIDE EFFECTS

- Tachycardia, premature ventricular contraction, hypotension
- Nausea, vomiting, water intoxication

NURSING IMPLICATIONS

1. Frequently assess baseline vital signs, blood pressure, and fetal heart rate.
2. Constantly monitor frequency, duration, and strength of contractions.
3. Stop the infusion; notify the HCP if the resting uterine pressure is greater than 15 to 20mm Hg, if contractions are lasting longer than 1 minute or if they are occurring more frequently than every 2 to 3minutes, or if an alteration in fetal heart rhythm or rate occurs.
4. Maintain input and output; evaluate for excessive water retention.
5. Do not confuse with vasopressin (Pitressin), which is an antidiuretic hormone.

Important nursing implications | Serious/life-threatening implications

Most frequent side effects | Patient teaching

Rh_o(D) IMMUNE GLOBULIN (RhIG) (RhoGAM)

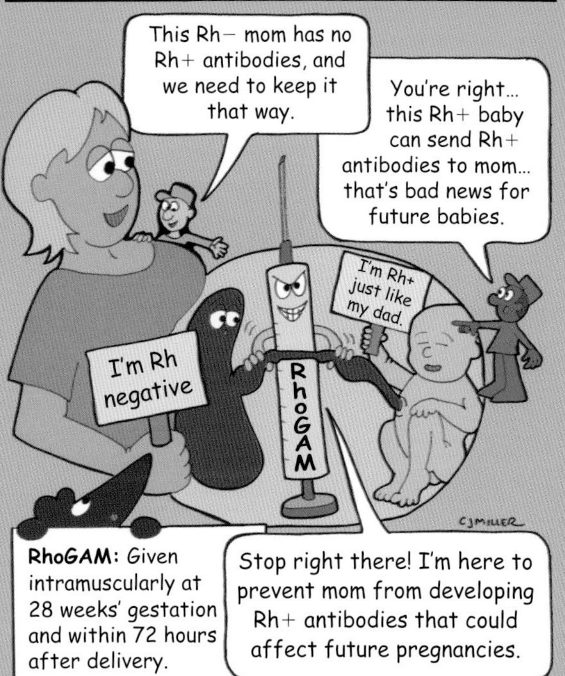

What You Need to Know

Rh_o(D) Immune Globulin (RhoGAM)

CLASSIFICATION

Immune globulin; immunosuppressant

ACTIONS

Rh_o(D) immune globulin is a concentrated immunoglobulin preparation that contains antibodies to Rh_o(D). These antibodies destroy any fetal red blood cells in the maternal circulation and prevent an Rh-negative woman from developing antibodies after exposure to Rh_o(D)-positive blood.

USES

- Prevents sensitization in the Rh-negative pregnant patient when given in the last trimester of pregnancy, as well as after abortion or miscarriage
- Following chorionic villus sampling, amniocentesis, percutaneous umbilical blood sampling, ectopic pregnancy, or any risk of fetal/maternal hemorrhage (trauma)

CONTRAINDICATIONS

- Not given to Rh-positive women
- Mother already has positive antibodies
- Allergic reaction to human immune globulin
- Not given to the newborn

SIDE EFFECTS

- Uncommon
- Slight temperature elevation and irritation at the injection site

NURSING IMPLICATIONS

1. Administered intramuscularly at 28 weeks' gestation and another dose if delivery does not occur within 12 weeks and within 72 hours after delivery.
2. May also be administered to Rh-negative women receiving a blood transfusion or who have had a spontaneous or induced abortion or amniocentesis.
3. Instruct Rh-negative patients to advise their HCP of their Rh-negative status.
4. Inject intramuscular preparation into deltoid or anterolateral aspect of the upper thigh; do not inject into the gluteal muscle.
5. Teach family how RhoGAM works, so they understand the importance of prenatal care and monitoring.

Important nursing implications | Serious/life-threatening implications

Most frequent side effects | Patient teaching

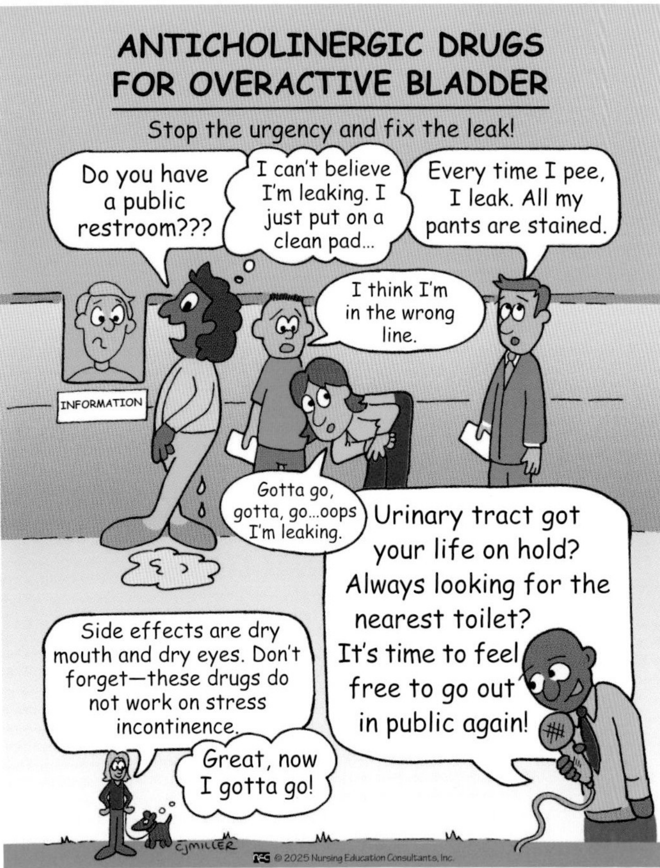
ANTICHOLINERGIC DRUGS FOR OVERACTIVE BLADDER
Stop the urgency and fix the leak!
Do you have a public restroom???
I can't believe I'm leaking. I just put on a clean pad...
Every time I pee, I leak. All my pants are stained.
I think I'm in the wrong line.
INFORMATION
Gotta go, gotta, go...oops I'm leaking.
Urinary tract got your life on hold? Always looking for the nearest toilet? It's time to feel free to go out in public again!
Side effects are dry mouth and dry eyes. Don't forget—these drugs do not work on stress incontinence.
Great, now I gotta go!
CJMILLER
© 2025 Nursing Education Consultants, Inc.

What You Need to Know

Anticholinergic Drugs for Overactive Bladder

EXAMPLES

Oxybutynin (Ditropan), solifenacin (VESIcare), tolterodine (Detrol), darifenacin (Enablex), festerodine (Toviaz), trospium (Sanctura XR)

CLASSIFICATION

Anticholinergic, muscarinic antagonists

ACTION

Block receptors in the bladder detrusor to relax bladder contractions.

USES

- To treat patients with an overactive bladder having symptoms of urinary frequency, urgency, or urge incontinence

PRECAUTIONS AND CONTRAINDICATIONS

- Combined use with other anticholinergic medications will intensify the side effects.
- Urinary retention, bladder obstruction, benign prostatic hypertrophy.

SIDE EFFECTS

- Dry mouth, dry eyes, blurred vision, constipation, gastric discomfort
- Oxybutynin: urinary retention and hesitancy; tachycardia more common; with transdermal preparations, pruritus at the application site
- Solifenacin: caution with cardiac patients with QT prolongation
- Tolterodine: has a short half-life, needs twice-a-day dosing; can prolong the QT interval

NURSING IMPLICATIONS

1. Monitor for incontinence and postvoid residuals.
2. Teach patient how to use saline eye drops if dry eyes are a problem.
3. Do not open or chew extended-release capsules.
4. Teach behaviors to modify incontinence problem:
   - Avoidance of caffeine
   - Pelvic floor muscle exercises (Kegel exercises)
   - Scheduled voiding times
   - Timing of fluid intake
5. Teach women the importance of using incontinence feminine pads and not a feminine pad for menstrual flow.

Important nursing implications | Serious/life-threatening implications

Most frequent side effects | Patient teaching

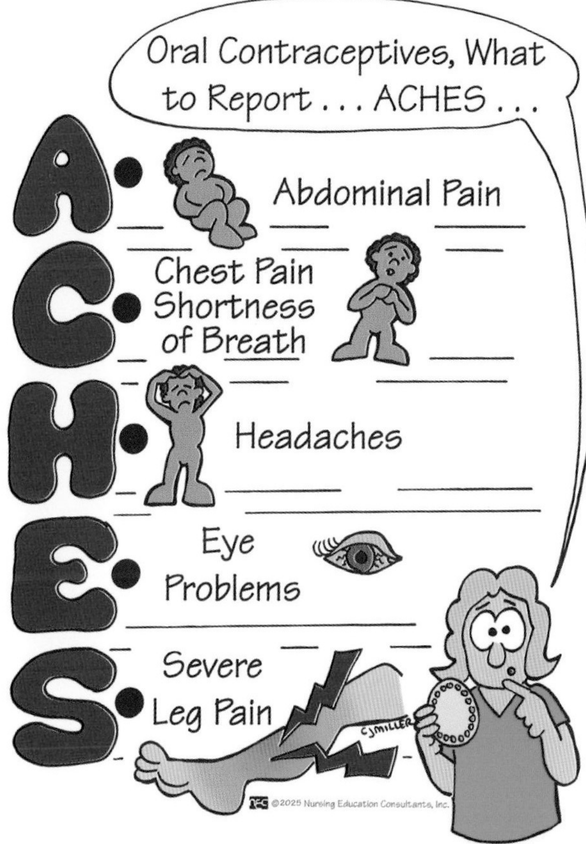

Oral Contraceptives, What to Report . . . ACHES . . .
A: Abdominal Pain
C: Chest Pain Shortness of Breath
H: Headaches
E: Eye Problems
S: Severe Leg Pain
CJMILLER
©2025 Nursing Education Consultants, Inc.

What You Need to Know

Oral Contraceptives: Serious Adverse Effects

ACTION ■ Black Box Warning

Combination of estrogen and progestin or progestin-only (minipill) inhibits ovulation

USES

- To prevent pregnancy

CONTRAINDICATIONS

- Pregnancy, history of thromboembolic disorders, cerebrovascular disease, coronary occlusion, breast cancer, abnormal liver function, abnormal vaginal bleeding, smokers older than 35 years

PRECAUTIONS

- Women who have diabetes, hypertension, cardiac disease, gallbladder problems, epilepsy, uterine leiomyoma, migraine headaches
- Women who are having surgery because immobilization will increase the risk of developing a postoperative thrombosis

SIDE EFFECTS

- Minor: breast tenderness, nausea, bloating, edema, weight gain
- Serious: increased blood pressure, right upper quadrant abdominal pain, chest pain, headaches, eye problems, severe leg pain

NURSING IMPLICATIONS

1. The patient can take oral contraceptives immediately after delivery for birth control if she is not breast-feeding.
2. Encourage an annual pelvic examination and Papanicolaou smear.
3. If patient is using a 28-day-cycle combination product (except Natazia) and misses a pill during the first week, take it as soon as possible and continue with the pack. If patient misses two doses during the second or third week, take one pill as soon as possible and continue with the active pills in the pack; skip the placebo pills and go straight to a new pack once the active pills have been taken. If patient misses three doses in the second or third week, follow the same instructions given for missing one or two pills and teach the patient to use another form of birth control during this time.
4. If patient is taking Natazia, have her consult the package insert or her HCP for directions to follow when a pill is missed.
5. The patient should take pills (particularly progestin-only) at the same time each day (e.g., with a meal, at bedtime). If a minipill (up to two of them) is missed, it should be taken immediately. If three pills are missed, then it should be stopped and resumed when menstruation occurs.

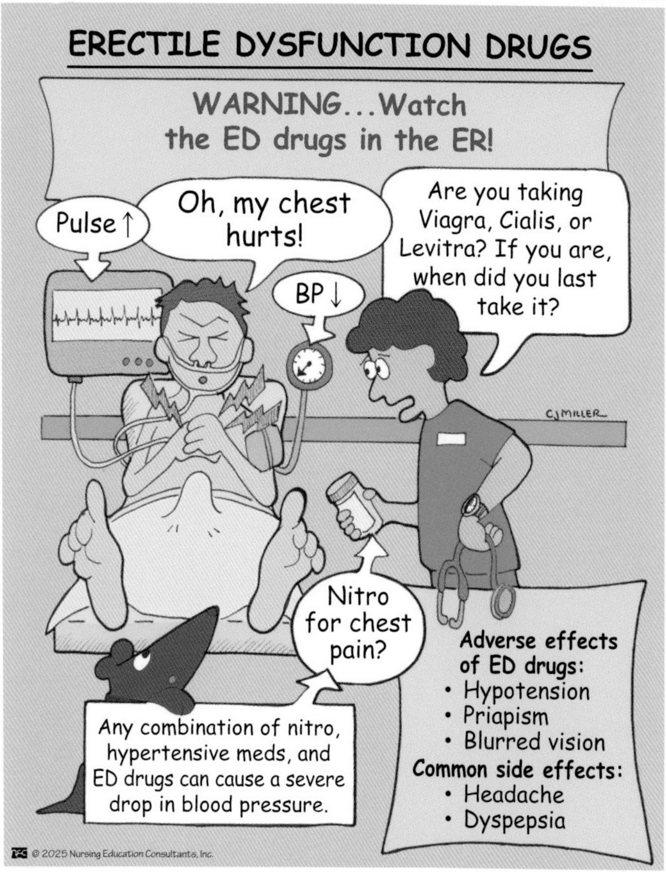

ERECTILE DYSFUNCTION DRUGS

WARNING...Watch the ED drugs in the ER!

Pulse ↑

Oh, my chest hurts!

BP ↓

Are you taking Viagra, Cialis, or Levitra? If you are, when did you last take it?

CJMILLER

Nitro for chest pain?

Any combination of nitro, hypertensive meds, and ED drugs can cause a severe drop in blood pressure.

Adverse effects of ED drugs:
- Hypotension
- Priapism
- Blurred vision

Common side effects:
- Headache
- Dyspepsia

What You Need to Know

Erectile Dysfunction Drugs

ACTIONS

Phosphodiesterase-5 inhibitors increase arterial pressure and reduce venous outflow in the penis, thereby causing engorgement to produce and/or enhance an erection. It only enhances the normal erectile response to sexual stimuli. In the absence of stimuli, no erection occurs.

USES

- Organic, psychogenic, mixed-cause origin of erectile dysfunction (ED)

CONTRAINDICATIONS AND PRECAUTIONS

- Do not take within 24 hours of taking nitrate medication.
- Patients taking alpha-blocker medications should avoid ED drugs.
- Avoid vardenafil (Levitra), but not sildenafil (Viagra) or tadalafil (Cialis) in men taking class I or class III antidysrhythmic drugs or drugs that prolong the QT interval.
- Dose may be reduced when patients take verapamil or diltiazem.

SIDE EFFECTS

- Severe hypotension when used within 24 hours of nitrates
- Dyspepsia, headache, nasal congestion
- Vardenafil: use caution with medications that cause a prolonged QT interval
- Erection lasting longer than 4 to 6 hours (priapism)

NURSING IMPLICATIONS

1. Instruct patients taking cardiac medications to consult with the HCP about the safe use of ED drugs.
2. Ask male patients who are complaining of chest pain if they have taken an ED drug within the last 48 hours.
3. ED drugs can be taken by men who are healthy enough for normal sexual activity.
4. Instruct patient to report erections lasting longer than 4 hours to the HCP.
5. Teach patient to report any sudden loss of vision in one or both eyes or sudden hearing loss.
6. Tadalafil has a 36-hour duration of action; other ED drugs have a 4-hour duration.

Important nursing implications | Serious/life-threatening implications

Most frequent side effects | Patient teaching

MEDICATION FOR BENIGN PROSTATIC HYPERPLASIA

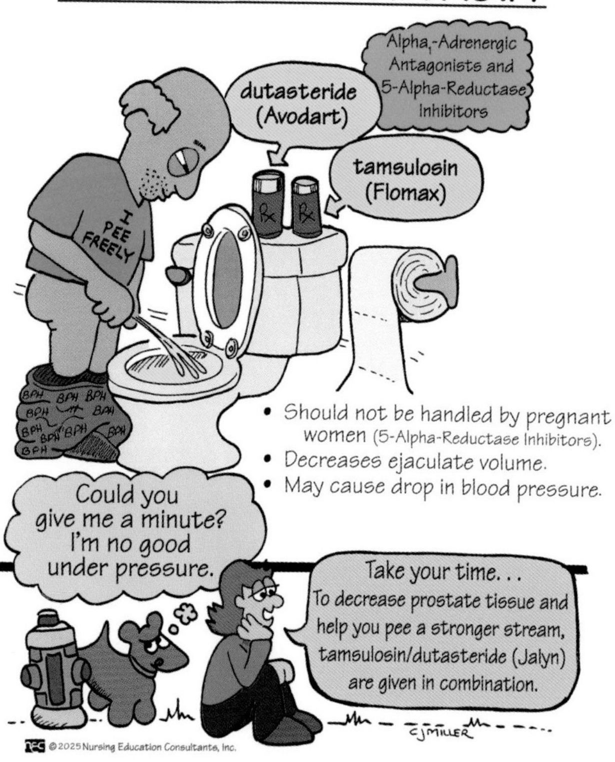

What You Need to Know

Drugs for Benign Prostatic Hyperplasia

EXAMPLES

Alpha$_1$-adrenergic antagonists: tamsulosin (Flomax), terazosin, alfuzosin (Uroxatral), doxazosin (Cardura), silodosin (Rapaflo). (*Note how the generic names end in "osin."*)
5-Alpha-reductase inhibitors: finasteride (Proscar) and dutasteride (Avodart). (*Note how the generic names end in "steride."*)

ACTIONS

- Alpha$_1$-adrenergic antagonists—block receptors that relax the smooth muscle of the bladder neck, thereby reducing the obstruction of the urethra. Do not decrease the size of the prostate. Action is rapid.
- 5-Alpha-reductase inhibitors—promote regression of the prostate tissue, thereby decreasing the obstruction of the urethra. Action is slow.
- Medications are frequently given together.

USES

Relieve urinary obstruction caused by benign prostatic hyperplasia

CONTRAINDICATIONS

Pregnancy and pediatrics

SIDE EFFECTS

- Finasteride—may decrease the level of prostate-specific antigen (PSA) marker for prostate cancer; decrease ejaculate volume, decrease libido
- Tamsulosin (Flomax) and terazosin—hypotension, fainting, dizziness, abnormal ejaculation

NURSING IMPLICATIONS

1. Pregnant women should not handle the 5-alpha-reductase inhibitors.
2. Before beginning finasteride therapy, the PSA value should be determined and reevaluated again 6 months after therapy begins.
3. Tamsulosin (Flomax) and terazosin—explain to patient that he should have less difficulty urinating within a few days of starting medication.
4. Finasteride (Proscar)—decrease in the prostatic tissue will take several months.

Important nursing implications | Serious/life-threatening implications
Most frequent side effects | Patient teaching

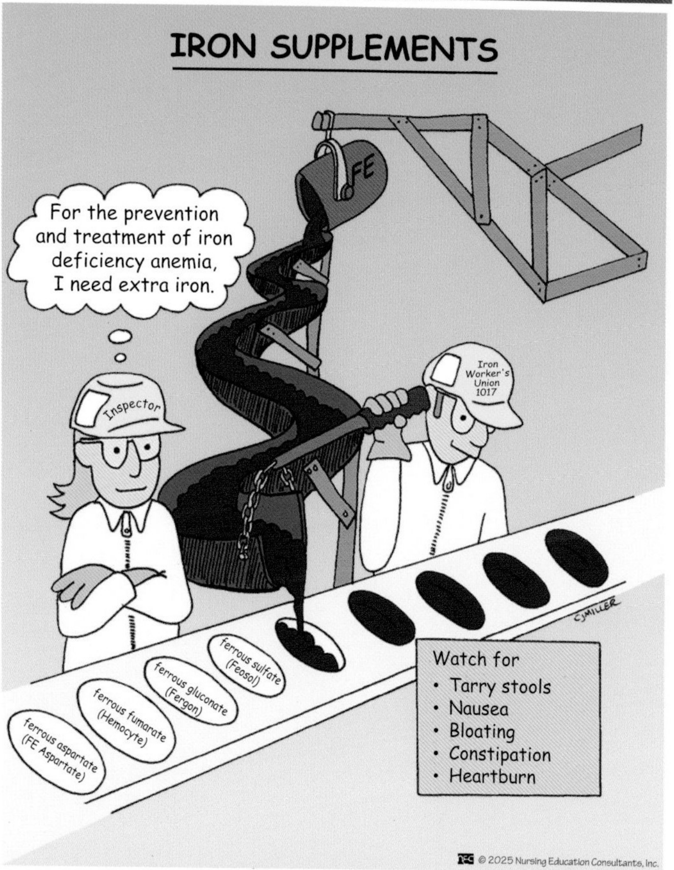

IRON SUPPLEMENTS

For the prevention and treatment of iron deficiency anemia, I need extra iron.

FE

Inspector

Iron Worker's Union 1017

ferrous sulfate (Feosol)

ferrous gluconate (Fergon)

ferrous fumarate (Hemocyte)

ferrous aspartate (FE Aspartate)

CJMILLER

Watch for
- Tarry stools
- Nausea
- Bloating
- Constipation
- Heartburn

What You Need to Know

Iron Supplements (Oral Ferrous Iron Salts)

ACTION

Hematinic agent used in the production of normal hemoglobin and red blood cells (RBCs) for transportation and utilization of oxygen.

USES

- Iron deficiency anemia
- Prophylactic use in pregnancy and childhood, and in women with menorrhagia

CONTRAINDICATIONS AND PRECAUTIONS

- All anemias other than iron deficiency anemia
- Peptic ulcers, regional enteritis, ulcerative colitis
- Iron-containing products are leading cause of iron poisoning in young children

SIDE EFFECTS

- Gastrointestinal (GI) disturbances—nausea (usually transient), heartburn (pyrosis), bloating, constipation
- Teeth staining, tarry stools or dark-green discoloration (not associated with bleeding)
- Iron toxicity due to accidental or intentional overdose (usually in children and not with therapeutic doses)

NURSING IMPLICATIONS

1. Do not give with antacids, calcium supplements, dairy products, tetracyclines, or crush or chew sustained-release medications.
2. Space doses evenly throughout the day to increase RBC production.
3. Take between meals to maximize uptake.
4. Because liquid preparations stain the teeth, use a straw or dilute the liquid; follow with rinsing the mouth.
5. Teach patient that oral iron supplements differ from one another and should not be interchanged.
6. Dietary teaching to include iron-rich foods—liver, eggs, red meats, fish, fowl.
7. Teach patient to store iron out of reach and in childproof containers; iron poisoning can be fatal to young children.
8. Parenteral deferoxamine (Desferal) and the oral drugs deferasirox (Exjade) and deferiprone (Ferriprox) are used for chronic iron overload caused by blood transfusions—drugs absorb iron and prevent toxic effects.

ORAL CALCIUM SUPPLEMENTS

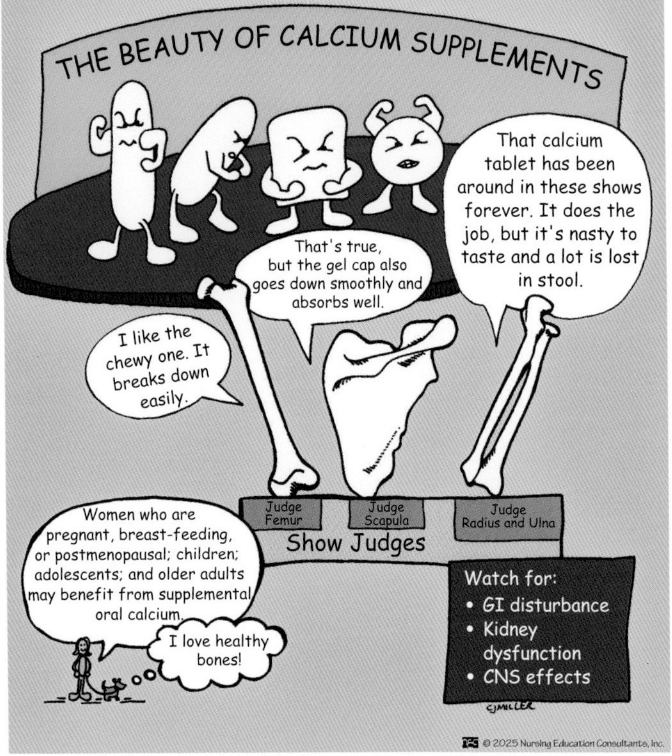

THE BEAUTY OF CALCIUM SUPPLEMENTS

That calcium tablet has been around in these shows forever. It does the job, but it's nasty to taste and a lot is lost in stool.

That's true, but the gel cap also goes down smoothly and absorbs well.

I like the chewy one. It breaks down easily.

Judge Femur

Judge Scapula

Judge Radius and Ulna

Show Judges

Women who are pregnant, breast-feeding, or postmenopausal; children; adolescents; and older adults may benefit from supplemental oral calcium.

I love healthy bones!

Watch for:
- GI disturbance
- Kidney dysfunction
- CNS effects

CJMILLER

What You Need to Know

Oral Calcium Supplements

CLASSIFICATION

Calcium salt

ACTION

Necessary for the normal functioning of the nervous, muscular, skeletal systems.

USES

- Treatment of mild hypocalcemia and taken as a dietary supplement
- Prophylactic for osteoporosis

CONTRAINDICATIONS AND PRECAUTIONS

- Hypercalcemia, hypophosphatemia, dehydration
- Presence or history of renal calculi or renal impairment

SIDE EFFECTS

- GI disturbances (nausea, vomiting, constipation)
- Kidney dysfunction (polyuria, stones)
- Central nervous system effects (lethargy, depression)
- Hypercalcemia—cardiac dysrhythmias and deposition of calcium into soft tissue

NURSING IMPLICATIONS

1. Encourage fluids with medication. Take with or after meals to promote absorption.
2. Increase fiber-containing foods to decrease constipation. Avoid foods that suppress calcium absorption—spinach, Swiss chard, beets, bran, whole-grain cereals.
3. Encourage patient to check with health care professional regarding calcium and cardiac medications.
4. Calcium carbonate has the highest percentage of calcium; however, calcium citrate preparations are more completely absorbed.
5. To maintain adequate absorption and decrease the loss of calcium, the patient should not take more than 600 mg at one time.
6. A calcium supplement is not a treatment for osteoporosis, but a preventive measure to promote bone health.
7. Advise patient against switching to different calcium preparations, as they differ with respect to amount of elemental calcium.

PYRIDOXINE (VITAMIN B_6) ISONIAZID (INH) AND LEVODOPA

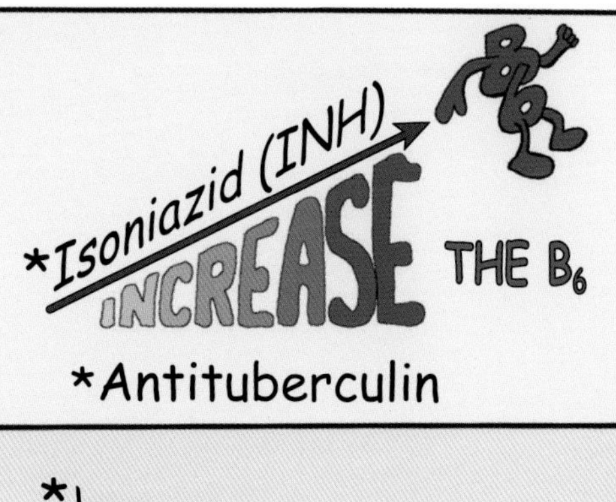

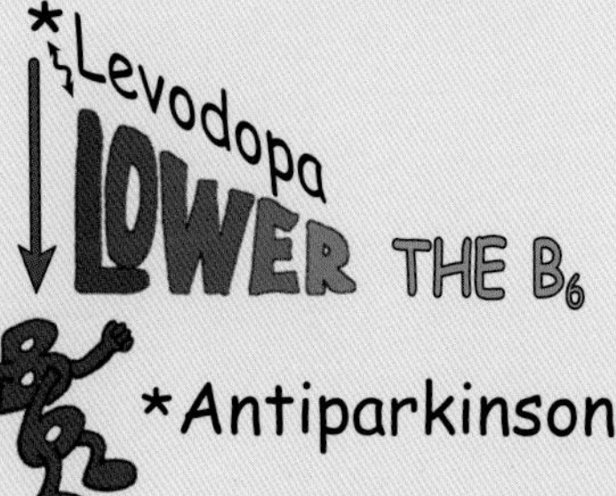

C.J. MILLER

What You Need to Know

Pyridoxine (Vitamin B_6): Isoniazid and Levodopa

CLASSIFICATION

Vitamin B_6 is a member of the vitamin B complex of water-soluble vitamins.

ACTION

Functions as a coenzyme in the metabolism of amino acids and proteins; it must be converted to an active form of pyridoxal phosphate.

DEFICIENCIES

- Common among patients with alcoholism.
- Isoniazid (INH) prevents conversion to active form.
- Symptoms of deficiency include peripheral neuritis, dermatitis, seborrheic dermatitis, depression, and confusion.

DRUG INTERACTIONS

- Vitamin B_6 interferes with the utilization of levodopa or carbidopa-levodopa, which are common medications in the treatment of Parkinson disease. Patients taking levodopa should not take vitamin B_6 supplements.

SIDE EFFECTS

- Extremely high dose: sensory neuropathy—ataxia and numbness to hands and feet

NURSING IMPLICATIONS

1. Patients taking INH need an increased intake of vitamin B_6 to prevent deficiency.
2. Patients taking levodopa need a decreased intake of vitamin B_6, which reverses the effects of the levodopa.
3. Evaluate nutritional adequacy.
4. Perform neurologic checks in the patient with vitamin B_6 issues.
5. Teach patient about dietary sources of vitamin B_6—meats and fish, especially organ meats; heavily fortified cereals; starchy vegetables; soy-based products.
6. Deficiency most often occurs in combination with deficiency of other B vitamins in patients who abuse alcohol.
7. To avoid neurologic injury, teach patient to consume no more than 100 mg/day of vitamin B_6.

Important nursing implications	Serious/life-threatening implications
Most frequent side effects	Patient teaching

CYANOCOBALAMIN
(Treatment of Vitamin B12 Deficiency)

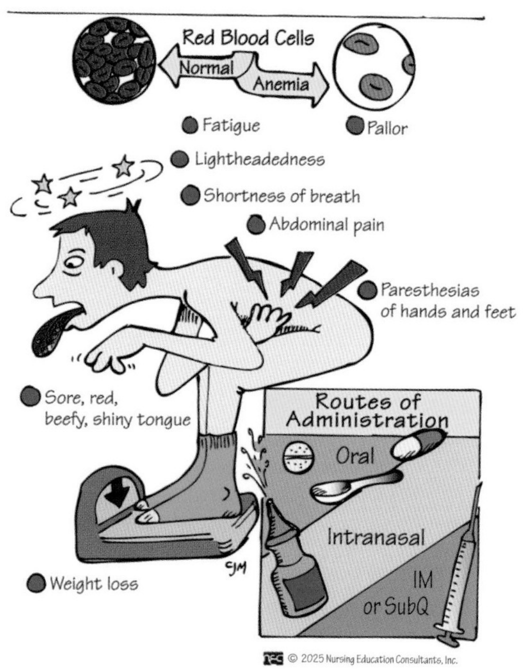

What You Need to Know

Cyanocobalamin (Vitamin B_{12})

ACTION

Hematinic agent used in the treatment of vitamin B_{12} deficiency. Most commonly, vitamin B_{12} deficiency is the result of impaired absorption due to regional enteritis, celiac disease, and development of antibodies against the intrinsic factor. Loss of the intrinisic factor from atrophy of gastric parietal cells and total gastric resection surgery leads to a deficiency state and syndrome called *pernicious anemia* (older term not used as often).

USES

- Vitamin B_{12} deficiency anemia (megaloblastic or macrocytic)
- Used in patients with increased B_{12} requirements (pregnancy, liver disease, hemorrhage, bariatric surgery, strict vegan diets)

CONTRAINDICATIONS AND PRECAUTIONS

- Hypersensitivity to cobalt, Leber disease
- Anemia and injury to the nervous system are main consequences of B_{12} deficiency
- When folic acid is combined with vitamin B_{12} to treat B_{12} deficiency, it is essential to monitor the dosage of B_{12} to be adequate because folic acid can mask continued B_{12} deficiency (by improving the hematologic picture), while allowing the neurologic consequences of B_{12} deficiency to progress

SIDE EFFECTS

- Hypokalemia may occur as a natural consequence of increased erythrocyte production
- Diarrhea, glossitis; generally devoid of serious adverse effects
- Pain at injection site

NURSING IMPLICATIONS

1. Administered either orally, intranasally, or by intramuscular or subcutaneous injection.
2. Oral therapy can be used for most patients.
3. Patients with severe neurologic impairment need parenteral administration.
4. Cyanocobalamin must NOT be given intravenously (IV).
5. Recovery from anemia occurs quickly (hematocrit level normal within 14–21 days); however, recovery from neurologic deficits is slow and complete recovery may never occur if treatment was delayed.
6. Teach patient who lacks the intrinsic factor that lifelong treatment is required.

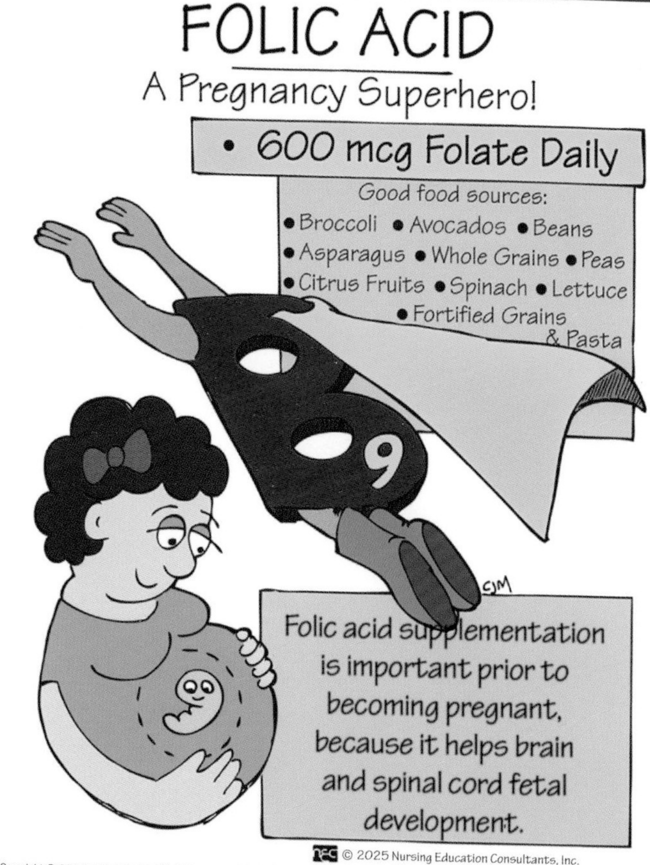

FOLIC ACID

A Pregnancy Superhero!

• 600 mcg Folate Daily

Good food sources:

- Broccoli
- Avocados
- Beans
- Asparagus
- Whole Grains
- Peas
- Citrus Fruits
- Spinach
- Lettuce
- Fortified Grains & Pasta

B9

SJM

Folic acid supplementation is important prior to becoming pregnant, because it helps brain and spinal cord fetal development.

What You Need to Know

Folic Acid

CLASSIFICATION

Vitamin B_9, water soluble.
Folate is the form in which the vitamin is found naturally in foods.
Folic acid is the form used to fortify grain products and other foods and vitamin supplements.

ACTIONS

Stimulates the production of platelets and RBCs in folate-deficiency anemia and is necessary for erythropoiesis and the formation of many coenzymes; crucial for proper brain function.

USES

- Incidence of neural tube defects, such as spina bifida and anencephaly, is decreased significantly with the daily intake of 600 mcg of supplemental folic acid prior to pregnancy; hence, all women capable of becoming pregnant should take supplemental 400 to 800 mcg of folic acid daily.
- Treatment of megaloblastic and macrocytic anemias due to folate deficiency.

CONTRAINDICATIONS

- None known

RECOMMENDED DIETARY ALLOWANCE

- Men and women aged 19 years and older should aim for 400 mcg daily.
- Pregnant women should take 600 mcg and lactating women require 500 mcg daily.
- People who regularly drink alcohol should aim for at least 600 mcg daily since alcohol can impair its absorption.

SIDE EFFECTS

- None known

NURSING IMPLICATIONS

1. Teach patients that they may take it without regard to food.
2. Teach patient to consume foods high in folic acid—beef liver (highest source of folate), citrus fruits, broccoli, spinach, asparagus, black-eyed peas, lettuce, beans, whole grains, avocados; fortified grains and pasta.
3. High intake of folate supplements might "mask" vitamin B_{12} deficiency to the point that some of the neurological problems become irreversible.

Important nursing implications | Serious/life-threatening implications
Most frequent side effects | Patient teaching

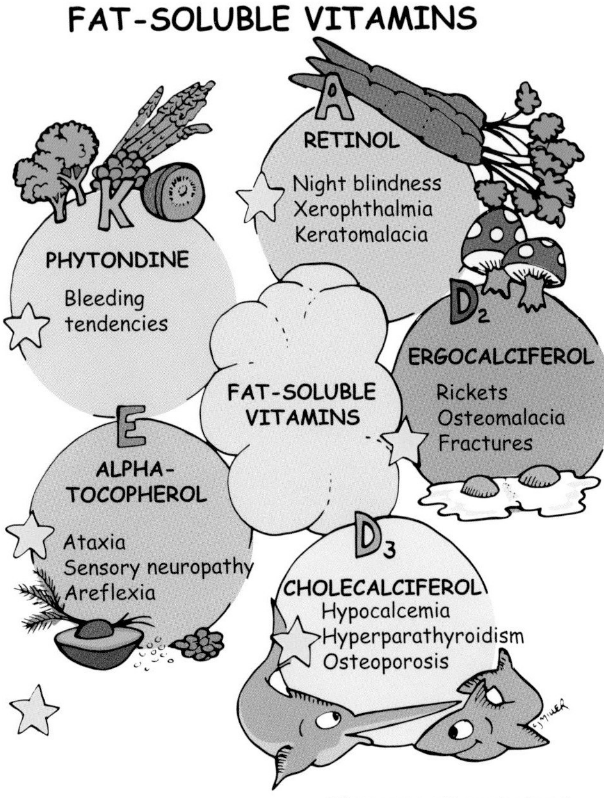
FAT-SOLUBLE VITAMINS
A
RETINOL
Night blindness
Xerophthalmia
Keratomalacia
K
PHYTONDINE
Bleeding
tendencies
FAT-SOLUBLE
VITAMINS
D2
ERGOCALCIFEROL
Rickets
Osteomalacia
Fractures
E
ALPHA-
TOCOPHEROL
Ataxia
Sensory neuropathy
Areflexia
D3
CHOLECALCIFEROL
Hypocalcemia
Hyperparathyroidism
Osteoporosis
© 2025 Nursing Education Consultants, Inc.

What You Need to Know

Fat-Soluble Vitamins (Vitamins A, D, E, K)

ACTION

Fat-soluble vitamins are absorbed in the small intestine and stored in the body's liver and adipose tissue. The four fat-soluble vitamins are vitamins A, D, E, and K. These vitamins are absorbed more easily by the body in the presence of dietary fat.

USES

- Vitamin A—helps support normal vision (especially at night); aids in immune function, growth and development, reproduction
- Vitamin D—aids in intestinal absorption of calcium to maintain healthy bones and in preventing rickets and osteomalacia
- Vitamin E—antioxidants aid in protecting cells and tissue from free radicals in environmental pollutants, pesticides, cigarette smoke
- Vitamin K—necessary for clot formation to stop bleeding; prophylactically given to prevent vitamin K deficiency bleeding in newborns

CONTRAINDICATIONS AND PRECAUTIONS

- Pregnancy (preformed vitamin A), bleeding disorders (vitamin E), elevated vitamin levels; vitamin toxicity
- Kidney and hepatic disease

SIDE EFFECTS

- Hypervitaminosis—jaundice, vomiting, skin changes (vitamin A)
- Dizziness, fatigue (vitamin D)
- Nausea, abdominal pain, fatigue, headache (vitamin E)
- Hematoma formation; pain at injection site (vitamin K)

NURSING IMPLICATIONS

1. Advise pregnant clients not to exceed upper limit and recommended dietary allowance for vitamin A, as it is a teratogenic that can cause fetal malformations and increase risk of hip fracture in patients.
2. To promote absorption, fat-soluble vitamins should be taken with food or milk products containing fat.
3. Teach patients not to take vitamin D supplements >4000 IU; may cause toxicity.
4. Advise patient that spending 10 to 15 minutes outside in the sun three times weekly (without sunscreen) can also aid in preventing vitamin D deficiency.
5. High doses of vitamin E may increase risk of heart failure and accelerate cancer progression.
6. Do not administer vitamin K (phytonadione) IV; may cause shock, cardiopulmonary arrest.

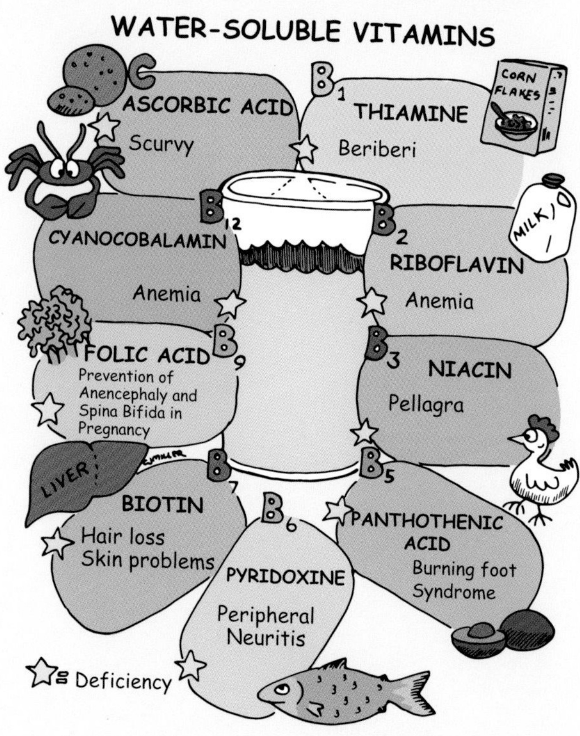
WATER-SOLUBLE VITAMINS
C
ASCORBIC ACID
Scurvy
B1
THIAMINE
Beriberi
CORN FLAKES
MILK
B12
CYANOCOBALAMIN
Anemia
B2
RIBOFLAVIN
Anemia
B9
FOLIC ACID
Prevention of
Anencephaly and
Spina Bifida in
Pregnancy
B3
NIACIN
Pellagra
LIVER
B7
BIOTIN
Hair loss
Skin problems
B6
PYRIDOXINE
Peripheral
Neuritis
B5
PANTHOTHENIC
ACID
Burning foot
Syndrome
= Deficiency
© 2025 Nursing Education Consultants, Inc.

What You Need to Know

Water-Soluble Vitamins (Vitamins B, C)

ACTION

Water-soluble vitamins are not stored in the body, as they are quickly absorbed in the body after ingestion and any excess is removed through urinary excretion. Vitamin B_{12} is the exception, as it can be stored in the liver. The water-soluble vitamins consist of vitamin C (*ascorbic acid*) and the B complex vitamins: B_1 (*thiamine*), B_2 (*riboflavin*), B_3 (*niacin*), B_5 (*pantothenic acid*), B_6 (*pyridoxine*), B_7 (*biotin*), B_9 (*folic acid*), B_{12} (*cobalamin*).

USES

- Vitamin C—promotes collagen production; assists in absorption of iron; prevention and treatment of scurvy.
- B complex vitamins are primarily indicated for prevention and treatment of vitamin deficiency.

CONTRAINDICATIONS AND PRECAUTIONS

- Kidney disease
- Hepatic disease
- Hypersensitivity
- Vitamin toxicity

SIDE EFFECTS

- Diarrhea, bright yellow urine (vitamin C)
- Flushing, tingling, itching of skin (niacin)
- Nausea, heartburn, photosensitivity (vitamin B_6)

NURSING IMPLICATIONS

1. Obtain a list of prescribed and over-the-counter medications that the patient is taking, as the B complex vitamins can interact with certain medications.
2. Ask patient if they are taking biotin before obtaining lab draws. Biotin can interfere with certain laboratory test results (may cause falsely low troponin results); this may lead to a missed diagnosis of heart attack.
3. To minimize GI discomfort, water-soluble vitamins can be taken with food.
4. Give patient aspirin 30 minutes prior to administering niacin to minimize flushing.

Index

Note: Page numbers followed by "*f*" indicate figures and "*t*" indicate tables.

–A–

–B–

–D–

–E–

-F-

-G-

H

—M—

—N—

-Q-

-R-

-S-

–T–

–U–

–V–

–W–

–X–

–Z–